Lose Weight Without Dieting

First Edition

PONCE INLET PRESS
Ponce Inlet, Florida

Optimal Health Protocols
311 Shady Place
Daytona Beach, Florida 32114
Telephone: 386-308-5395

Copyright © 2009 by W.G. Miller

All rights reserved. No part of this book may be reproduced or utilized in any form or by any means, electronic or mechanical, including photocopying, recording, or by any information storage and retrieval system, without permission in writing from the publisher.

Disclaimer: *This book is intended as an informational guide. The remedies, approaches, and techniques described herein are meant to supplement, and not to be a substitute for, professional medical care or treatment. They should not be used to treat a serious ailment without prior consultation with a qualified health care professional.*

This book is dedicated to all the overweight people that struggle daily with their efforts to lose their excess weight while being ridiculed and tormented by the rest of society. Now you can lose the weight you have so desired to lose and finally be happy and at peace with yourselves!

Contents

2	Introduction	
4	Chapter 1:	The "Popular" Diets & Why They May Not Have Worked For You
10	Chapter 2:	Getting Off The Weight-Gain, Weight-Loss Rollercoaster
13	Chapter 3:	The Science of Weight Loss
46	Chapter 4:	The Psychology of Weight Loss
54	Chapter 5:	The New Menu
83	Chapter 6:	Supplements for Sustained Health
129	Chapter 7:	Exercise: The Fountain of Youth
136	Chapter 8:	How Much Water is the Right Amount?
140	Chapter 9:	What the Future Holds
144	Appendix 1:	Meal Suggestions
163	Appendix 2:	Recommended Reading
164	About the Author	
166	Bibliography	

"If we could give every individual the right amount of nourishment and exercise, not too little and not too much, we would have found the safest way to health."

—**Hippocrates c. 460 – 377 B.C.**

Introduction

According to the latest statistics from the third National Health and Nutrition Examination Survey (NHANES), 97 million Americans are overweight or obese.[1] There are an estimated 300 million people in the United States, resulting in a relative number of one in three Americans being overweight or obese.

Excess weight is often accompanied by high blood pressure, high blood cholesterol, type 2 diabetes, coronary heart disease, certain types of cancer, stroke, arthritis, breathing problems, and psychological disorders, such as depression, not to mention other health problems. The total costs attributed to obesity-related disease surpass $100 billion annually in the United States.[2]

Weight loss is not just a matter of wanting to look and feel better, it is a necessity if you want to get and stay healthy and let's face it, who doesn't.

The prevalence of obesity in children has increased markedly, with approximately 20% - 25% of children either overweight or obese.[3] An estimated 25.6% of adults in the United States reported being obese in 2007, an increase of nearly 2 percent since 2005 according to the Office of the Surgeon General. The economic cost of obesity in the United States was estimated to be $117 billion in 2000.[4]

---

[1] http://win.niddk.nih.gov/statistics/
[2] http://health.nytimes.com/health/guides/specialtopic/weight-management/print.html
[3] http://www.medicinenet.com/obesity_weight_loss/article.htm
[4] http://www.thecommunityguide.org/obesity/index.html

Based on national survey data collected between 1988 and 1994 by the Office of the Surgeon General, The prevalence of overweight and obesity increases until about age 60, after which time it begins to decline.[5] Obesity is also increasing rapidly throughout the world, and the incidence of obesity nearly doubled form 1991 to 1998.[6]

"Overweight" was defined as a body mass index (BMI) of 25 to 29.9 kg/m^2 and obesity as a BMI of 30 kg/m^2.[7] BMI will be further defined later so don't concern yourself with it at this time. The bottom line is, if you are overweight and you know it, you probably don't need to prove you are overweight or need to know just how overweight the government thinks you are statistically.

Obviously, you understand that there is a problem and you purchased this book to solve it so let's get on with it.

---

[5] http://www.surgeongeneral.gov/topics/obesity/calltoaction/fact_glance.htm

[6] http://www.prlog.org/10335113-obesity-global-epidemic-and-overweight-and-obesity-issues-solved-only-aastha-healthcare.html

[7] *Nutrition Secrets*, by Charles W. Van Way, Carol S. Ireton-Jones - 2004 - Medical - 284 pages

Chapter 1: The "Popular" Diets & Why They May Not Have Worked For You

How many times have you started that new diet all excited, convinced that this one is it; This is the diet that is finally going to get you down to your "target" weight and keep you there. But each time the same thing happens. You may lose all the weight you want to lose, or almost all of it, and then you start cheating a little and then a lot and pretty soon you are off the diet and back to the weight you started at plus a little more which you attribute to the stress of being on the diet in the first place.

One thing you probably noticed about these diets was that you generally had to either eat really small portions or you were limited to very bland, "rice cake" type food. One diet program advertised on television says that you can even eat chocolate cake and then they show you the piece of cake. It looks very tasty but it's probably about one inch square. Ever noticed they never lay a fork next to the plate? There's a good reason for that. The fork would look like a giant pitchfork because the piece of cake is so small. Come on, that's not a piece of cake! That's a sample of cake but not even close to a piece of cake. They also show you on the same advertisement a hamburger on a bun and other foods that are, not only not that healthy for you, but are certainly not something you would want to be eating if you are trying to lose weight.

The bottom line with these diets is that they don't work for most people. The main reason is that the hardest thing to do when you are wanting to diet is to go hungry. I remember when I was in wrestling in high school and I had to lose weight by Friday in order to wrestle in an upcoming meet. I would starve myself for two or three days, lose 10 or 11 pounds and wrestle for six minutes on Friday. First of all, let me be the first to say, if I tried to do that today it would probably kill me. It is amazing what your body can take when you are young and healthy.

The most difficult part of this whole dieting thing, which is the point of all this, was going hungry. It affected how I slept, my ability to concentrate, my mood and energy levels and my overall ability to think and react. There was nothing in my life that was not affected by the hunger, and all in a negative way I might add.

The only positive thing that came out it was that I lost the weight and got to wrestle in the meet on Friday. Other than that, it was awful! I would have to go back and re-read chapters I had already read because I couldn't remember the information I had read when I was so hungry. My lack of concentration and focus during the intense dieting periods had rendered me almost totally ineffective at things I did normally with ease.

This is the reason I think most diets fail, because they cause you to go hungry which upsets every other aspect of your life. It even causes you to be ineffective in some normal, everyday facets of life and have to do tasks two and three times to get them done, all because you are preoccupied with hunger.

This frustration causes stress and eventually you stop this damn diet and get back to normal!

Most diets predispose you to failure for two different reasons. One type of diet gives you great tasting, fattening foods but only small tiny, tiny little portions. The other type of diet lets you have as much celery and rice cakes as you want. Guess how much celery and rice cakes I want? If you said none, you already know me pretty well. Even if I haven't eaten all day I still don't think a rice cake is tasty or satisfying. I couldn't care less that I can have as much of that crap as I want. I don't want any of it!

What you will begin to learn in a few pages is how you can lose weight eating tasty, healthy foods and not have to limit the quantity and go hungry, within reason of course.

The reason I say, "within reason" is because if you weigh 900 pounds and you eat 17 bologna sandwiches for lunch every day, you must reduce the quantity of food you eat if you expect to lose weight. By the same token, if you weigh 900 pounds, you need to be under the care of a physician and not reading this book. For the rest of us, cutting out fattening food most of the time will be a big part of eliminating the excess weight you are carrying around.

If you get on one of these diets where you have to buy all your food from some company, then how are you ever going to eat at a restaurant? What are you going to do on holidays? What are you going to do when someone invites you over to their house for dinner? You certainly cannot bring your little microwave diet dinner with you; People would think you were nuts.

All of these situations occur in all of our lives and in all of these cases we have to go off the diet for these meals if we are on one of the diets where we buy special food. These diets do not teach you how to eat healthy in the real world and as soon as you quit buying this special, expensive food, you begin to gain back all the weight you lost.

If you are cheating on these meals then why not cheat a lot and have desert and everything? Then you get back on the scale and you realize you have gained back all the weight you lost in the previous week after suffering through a painful and debilitating starvation diet period.

I wanted to briefly outline why these diets fail so you would realize you are not alone. If the last few pages read like your biography there's a reason. Everyone, or almost everyone, goes through this same rollercoaster ride year after year and diet after diet.

We have our fat clothes and our skinny clothes. We get skinny then something traumatic happens and there we are with Twinkies and potato chips eating away the frustration and digging out our fat clothes from the back of the closet.

Let's get on to what works and why so you can begin to reach your goals. This time, as you lose the weight, throw out your fat clothes! You will not need them anymore! You are going to learn how to get the weight off, how to eat out at restaurants correctly, how to eat holiday meals correctly, how to accept dinner invitations and eat correctly and how to become thin and healthy for the rest of your life. In addition, you will learn the all important, "how and when to cheat." Let's face it you can't restrict the type and amount of food you eat every single meal, week after week and year after year so you need to know how to cheat without discouraging yourself from continuing with the weight loss.

This method does not require you to never cheat. You can cheat. Just go right back to the foods that keep the weight off. If your skinny clothes begin to get a little snug, go back to the basics you are getting ready to learn in a few pages and off comes those few pounds that caused the clothes to get a little too snug and you're back to thin and healthy once again.

Once you learn how this all works and you realize how much better you feel, you will become very adamant about sticking to the foods that keep the weight off and avoiding the foods that put it back on. You will notice that the foods you thought you liked so much actually make you feel sluggish and tired, even a little sick.

Many people even report that after a long time without these foods, re-introducing them into their diet, even temporarily, caused indigestion and nausea. It is a little disappointing when this happens but keep in mind you are changing both physically and mentally and the way you view all food is also changing. Don't deny the change or be disappointed when your favorite food, or what you thought was your favorite food, makes you feel ill and eventually doesn't even sound good anymore. The changes in the way you view these foods is evidence you are making permanent life changes that will keep you thin for the rest of your life.

Chapter 2: Getting Off The Weight-Gain, Weight-Loss Rollercoaster

Even though most diets don't generally work in the long run, you continue to search for the one that will. Because of the extra stress that most "diets" cause in your life, you tend to not just gain back the weight you lost in the short time you were on the diet, but as a result of the added stress of being on the diet you gain a little extra. So now you have a little more weight you want to lose and you feel like a failure. You wait a while and then you hear about or read about a diet that the stars in Hollywood are having great success with. Now it's time to try another fad diet and drop another few temporary pounds.

If this cycle has been repeating over and over throughout your life, you're not alone. Most people with a weight problem have it for many years and in many cases they die overweight having never succeeded in their life long desire to lose the excess pounds. Gaining and losing this excess weight repeatedly is extremely unhealthy and causes loads of stress on your organs and your body as a whole.

It doesn't have to be that way anymore. What you are getting ready to learn is not a diet but a **"New Menu."** As mentioned earlier, diets generally either limit the amounts of real tasty food that you can eat or allow an unlimited amount of rice cakes or some other dreadfully bland, "almost-not-even food" choices.

The **New Menu** that we are getting ready to show you consists completely of healthy, tasty foods. There is nothing on the list that is unhealthy for you or bland tasting. So let's get started with the good news. We are going to show you how you can lose weight and not have to eat bland food or limit the amount of food you eat, within reason. Maybe that sounds too good to be true but for once, it's not!

Now, before we outline the actual menu you will be changing to, we need to take a look at the science of dieting and the psychology behind actually losing the weight and keeping it off. It is important to learn the science behind dieting so you understand how this all works and are not just taking my word for it. Not only that but once you truly understand why the weight has been so difficult to lose you will be better equipped to lose the weight and keep it off. You will understand why the other diets failed you and begin realizing that maybe; just maybe it wasn't your fault. Maybe you were just listening to the wrong people.

Along with the science of dieting, the psychology behind weight loss is equally important. You need to be fully committed to losing the weight and in order to do so you must be totally convinced that you can and will lose the excess weight. Without this belief the rest of the program will not work so it is paramount that you believe that you will lose the weight.

You must begin to see yourself as the thin person you are striving for. We will also help you eliminate the triggers that have caused you to over eat in the past. If these triggers are not removed and replaced with correct thinking you will end up back on the rollercoaster. You certainly want to stop the viscous cycle of losing weight and then letting these negative triggers cause you to eat the wrong foods and re-gain the weight you have just lost.

Chapter 3: The Science of Weight Loss

Trying to lose weight without truly understanding what is going on specifically is close to impossible. You follow along with a diet and as soon as you notice one little thing that doesn't seem to work you immediately suspend your belief that the diet will work and that you will lose the weight you desire to lose. This is precisely why it is so important to understand what is really going on. This allows you to understand and even predict the things you are feeling as you begin to lose the excess weight.

Once you start to feel healthy and energetic by switching your menu and eating healthy, you will begin to realize that you are now providing your body with the health and nutrition it needs and wants. You will feel the difference and because of this chapter, you will also understand what is going on and why you are feeling the changes in your health and metabolism. As your health and ultimately your life changes, you will realize why the changes are occurring and you will understand the ill feelings you get when you cheat.

I never thought this would happen but sure enough after three months without any bread or potatoes I ate a half of a loaf of bread in three short days. I looked forward to that bread for over a week, toasted sourdough bread with butter. I could just taste it. When I did finally buy it and eat it I felt sluggish and almost ill for about 5 days. That is, the three days it took me to consume the half of a loaf of sourdough bread and the two days following the binge until that garbage had been eliminated from my system.

Your Metabolism and the Basal Metabolic Rate

Your metabolism is essentially the sum total of all the calories you consume and burn throughout the day. Your BMR or *Basal Metabolic Rate* is simply the energy you would expend if you laid around all day not moving or doing anything. Everyone's BMR is different and everyone's metabolism is different but there are a few elements that are the same. That is, we all process our food in the same biochemical way. This is providing, of course, that you do not have some debilitating illness which alters these processes. If this is the case consult your doctor before you begin any weight loss program. Assuming you are not one of these people let's continue.

In order to get a handle on your metabolism you need to get familiar with the amount of calories you are consuming each day and the amount you are burning each day also. After all it is the difference between these two numbers that determine whether you gain weight, lose weight or maintain your current weight. Counting calories is a drag so plan to do it only for a short time. After that you will begin to develop more of a "feel" for calories. You will know before you look up a particular food item whether it is high in calories or not. You will also be able to tell when you eat something whether it is high in calories or not. You will begin to associate the high calorie foods with that bloated, sluggish feeling accompanied by indigestion and gas and the low calorie foods with being alert, healthy and energetic.

A friend of mine who has asthma and allergies and has had them since he was a young boy adopted this new menu to see what it would do for him. He had a few extra pounds he wanted to get rid of and wanted to see if I knew what I was talking about. He called me on the third day after switching to the new menu and told me that he had laid down to go to bed and for the first time he could remember he was not wheezing. He also reported that he had slept sounder than normal and had awoken much more alert than normal.

There are many calorie counting tools available out there and even a few that are free. One that I found extremely useful even though it does require you to register is **My Calorie Counter** which can be found at: http://www.my-calorie-counter.com. Once you register you have access to many useful tools to help you reach your diet goals and help you track your progress along the way. Most importantly, at the beginning, when you don't have a clue about calories you can look up something like 45,000 different foods and find out their calorie content.

Once you get into the **New Menu** that will be presented in later chapters you will understand why it works so well. You end up getting full on healthy low calorie foods. The supplements you will learn about will create a continuous cleansing of your organs, especially your colon, where weight is often stored as "sludge" lining the walls of the colon. Naturally, getting rid of this sludge will certainly lower your weight. Preventing it from returning will certainly help in keeping your weight down.

You will see as you progress through this book that achieving weight loss and maintaining that weight loss is a result of many factors all of which play a role in getting and keeping you thin. The nice thing about there being multiple factors is that you don't have to do any of them perfect all the time. So long as you do most of them most of the time you will lose the weight you want to lose and be able to keep it off.

For now, I do want you to become very familiar with food and the amount of calories they add to your intake each day. This information will be in the back of your mind as you begin to look at all foods differently than you ever have before. The foods you once loved will begin to not seem so good because you will remember how they make you feel. Foods that maybe seemed plain will begin to have more flavor than you ever realized. I never realized how sweet fresh green beans are when you steam them and serve them with a little olive oil and sea salt and pepper. They taste absolutely fantastic! In the past I always thought they needed cream sauce or cheese sauce to make them complete. They just didn't seem finished without something else added. Now it seems like cream sauce or cheese sauce would ruin the flavor of the fresh beans. I noticed I could skin a whole bag of carrots, cut them up and steam them in about 30 minutes and then eat them at 4 different meals during the week along with other vegetables I had steamed on other days. More about this when we get into the actual menu and you begin taking the weight off and restoring the energy back into your life.

Zigzagging Calories

Zigzagging Calories simply means that you give your body different amounts of calories each day of the week and if you were to graph the number of calories over the week it would draw a zigzag pattern. This just means you start with the number of calories you want to consume each day, probably somewhere between 2000 and 2500 per day. You do that for one day then you eat slightly below this number of calories the next day. On the third day you eat more calories than you did on the first day and on the fourth day you eat the same as you did on the first day. The fifth day you eat the same as you did on the second day, the sixth day the same as on the third and finally on the seventh day you eat the same as you did on the first and fourth days.

This, presumably, causes the body to burn more calories than sticking with the same number of calories each day. Keeping everything the same every day causes your body to adapt and since you might be eating less calories your body may decide it needs to hang on to some of that extra weight to ward of the impending starvation. See the chart below for an example of zigzagging calories.

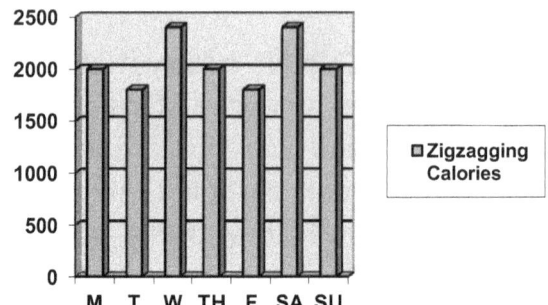

The Glycemic Index (GI) and the Glycemic Load (GL)

The Glycemic index measures how quickly blood sugar rises after you consume a particular amount and type of food. Therefore, the quicker a food is broken down to glucose, the quicker the blood sugar rises. This is true for most simple carbohydrates and almost, if not all, processed foods. Glucose is then actively transported across the cell membrane by insulin where it is used for energy in the mitochondria of the cell.

As *glycolysis* proceeds, *pyruvate* is produced. *Pyruvate* is either oxidized and enters *Kreb's Cycle* where it generates 29 *ATPs* or it is anaerobically (without oxygen) converted to lactic acid. *ATP* or *Adenosine Triphosphate* is what your body uses for energy. Note here that *Kreb's Cycle* actually generates 31 *ATPs* but it uses 2 in the process for a net total of 29 ATPs.

Simple carbohydrates and sugars as well as highly processed foods put a strain on the beta cells of your pancreas which produces the insulin required for active transport of the glucose across the cell membrane. If you eat food that converts to glucose quickly it causes the pancreas to work overtime to produce all of the insulin that is needed to transport the excess glucose across the cell membrane. Once all the glucose is transported across the cell membrane you experience what is referred to as "low-blood sugar" which over time can lead to hypoglycemia and type 2 diabetes.

A much better idea is to eat foods that convert slowly and steadily to glucose keeping a steady flow of insulin production by the pancreas and a steady amount of glucose being actively transported across the cell membrane.

Many studies have shown that diets utilizing foods with a low glycemic index work much better than diets containing foods with higher glycemic indices. This is at least part of what we are going to show you in a few chapters that will allow you to eat tasty foods and not have to go hungry to lose weight.

The glycemic index is measured on a scale from 0 to 100, where 100 is the rate at which pure glucose enters the bloodstream. A food with a glycemic index of 50 will raise blood sugar approximately half as much as pure glucose. Foods with a glycemic index of 50 or below are considered to be low on the glycemic index.

Problems with the glycemic index approach to dieting was realized when foods high on the glycemic index did not actually cause blood sugar to rise significantly. It seems that some foods that are listed as high on the glycemic index charts may not contain that much of the carbohydrate that causes this high glycemic index rating. Carrots are just such a food. While high on the glycemic index they do not cause a significant rise in blood sugar since they do not contain much of the carbohydrate that causes carrots to have this high glycemic index. This discrepancy was addressed with the introduction of the *Glycemic Load* (GL).

The *glycemic load* is the actual amount of carbohydrate in a specific type and quantity of food. Unlike the glycemic index, the glycemic load is computed by measuring the amount of carbohydrate in a food multiplied by the serving size. Foods with a glycemic load of less than 10 are considered to have a low glycemic load.

Some interesting comparisons ensue such as the fact that raw fruit has a lower GI and GL than the juice of the same fruit. Most fruits have a low GI but even watermelon with a high GI has a low GL.

Glycemic Index List

The following lists show the glycemic index (GI) and glycemic load (GL) for many foods. Make sure to note how high the glycemic index and glycemic load is for foods that are not on the **New Menu**.

Sugars

Glucose 85-111, average 100
Glucose consumed with 15-20 grams of fiber 57-85
Glucose consumed with protein and fat 56
Honey 32-87, average 55
Lactose 46
Table Sugar 68

Dairy Products

Milk, regular (full fat) 11-40, average 27
Milk, skim - 32
Yogurt w/o added sugar - 14-23

Starchy Vegetables

Beets 64
Carrots 16-92 average 47
Corn 37-62, average 53
Parsnips 97
Peas, green, fresh or frozen 39-54, average 48
Potato 56-111 - most averages usually given in high 80's

Potato, instant - 74-97, average 80
Rutabaga 72
Sweet potato - 44-78, average 61*

Sweet potatoes and yams cover a wide variety of species that are called different things in different places around the world. For example, garnet yams in the US are a type of sweet potato. Species are seldom given in the tables.

Legumes

Unless otherwise noted, "legumes" refer to dried beans or peas which are boiled. When canned beans are tested they tend to have a higher glycemic index.

Black-eyed peas 33-50
Butter beans 28-36, average 31
Chick peas (garbanzo beans) 31-36
Chick peas, canned 42
Kidney beans 13-46, average 34
Kidney beans, canned 52
Lentils 18-37
Lentils, canned 52
Navy beans (white beans, haricot) 30-39
Navy beans, pressure cooked 29-59
Peas, dried, split 32
Pinto beans 39
Pinto beans, canned 45
Soy beans 15-20
Soy beans, canned 14

Fruits

Apples - 28-44, average 38
Apricots, raw - 57
Apricots, canned in light syrup - 64
Apricots, dried 31
Apricot fruit spread (low sugar) - 55
Banana, under ripe - 30
Banana, overripe - 52
Banana, not specified 46-70
Cantaloupe 65
Cherries 22
Dates 103
Grapefruit 25
Grapes 46-49
Kiwi Fruit 47-58
Mangoes 41-60, average 51
Oranges 31-51, average 42
Papayas 56-60, average 59
Peaches 28-56
Pears 33-42
Pineapple 51-66
Plums 24-53
Raisins 64
Strawberries 40
Watermelon 72

Fruit Juice

Carrot Juice - 43
Cranberry Juice Cocktail - 52-68
Grapefruit Juice 48
Orange Juice 46-53
Pineapple Juice - 46
Tomato Juice - 38

Bread

White bread 64-87 - averages 70 and 73

Muffins, Cakes, Pancakes, Waffles Etc.

Whole wheat bread made with whole wheat flour - 52-87 average 71
Wheat bread made with 50% cracked wheat kernels 58
Wheat bread made with 75% cracked wheat kernels 48
Vary widely (38-102), but most between 55 and 80

Crackers

Rice Cakes - 61-91, average 78
High fiber rye crisp bread - 59-69, average 64
Stoned Wheat Thins - 67

Cold Cereal

All-Bran - 30-51, average 42
Bran Buds - 58
Bran Buds with Psyllium - 47
Cornflakes 72-92, average 81 (USA cornflakes were the 92)
Corn Chex 83
Crispix 87
Fruit Loops - 69
Golden Grahams - 71
Grape Nuts 67-85 average 71
Life - 66
Puffed Wheat - 67-80
Rice Krispie type cereals - 81-95
Rice Chex - 89
Shredded Wheat - 67-83 average 75
Special K - 54-84
Total - 76
Weetabix and similar - 61-74 - average 70

Hot Cereal

Cream of Wheat - 66
Instant Cream of Wheat - 74
Oatmeal from rolled oats (not instant) 42-75, the highest was US oatmeal average 58
Quick cooking oats - 66

Grains - Boiled Whole unless stated otherwise

Barley - 22-48
Barley, cracked - 50
Barley, rolled - 66
Buckwheat - 49-63
Cornmeal boiled in water - 69
Couscous (processed wheat) - 61-69
Millet - 71
Rice, long-grained white - 50-64, average 56
Rice, short and medium grained white - 83-93
Rice, brown - 66-87
Wheat, whole kernels - 30-48
Wheat, bulgar (cracked wheat) - 46-53, average 48

Pasta

The glycemic index of pasta made from wheat (most pasta) depends a lot upon the shape of the pasta (the thicker, the lower the GI), and the way it is cooked.

When cooked as the Italians do, "al dente" - somewhat firm - it has the lowest glycemic index. The longer you cook it, the softer it is, and the higher the GI. With variation depending upon these factors, most of the studies of wheat pasta show GIs in the 40's to low 60's, with a few dipping into the 30's.

Rice pasta (including brown) 40-92
Mung bean noodles (bean thread) 26-39

Nuts and Snack Foods

Cashews 22
Corn chips 72
Ice Cream - 37-80
Peanuts 7-23, average 14
Popcorn 55-89
Pop Tarts 70
Potato chips 51-57

Candy

Jelly Beans 76-80
Kudos Chocolate Chip Snack Bar 62
Life Savers 70
Mars Bar 62-68
Skittles 70
Snickers average 55

Soft Drinks

Coca Cola - 53-63 average 58
Gatorade - 78
Orange Soda - 68

Glycemic Load

The following table contains many common foods with their glycemic load and average serving size.

FOOD	Serving size (grams)	Glycemic load/serving
BAKERY PRODUCTS AND BREADS		
Banana cake, made with sugar	80	18
Banana cake, made without sugar	80	16
Sponge cake, plain	63	17
Vanilla cake made from packet mix with vanilla frosting (Betty Crocker)	111	24
Apple pie, made with sugar	60	13
Apple pie, made without sugar	60	9
Waffles, Aunt Jemima (Quaker Oats)	35	10
Bagel, white, frozen	70	25
Baguette, white, plain	30	15
Coarse barley bread, 75%-80% kernels, average	30	7
Hamburger bun	30	9
Kaiser roll	30	12

Pumpernickel bread	30	6
50% cracked wheat kernel bread	30	12
White wheat flour bread	30	10
Wonder™ bread, average	30	10
Whole-wheat bread, average	30	9
100% Whole Grain™ bread (Natural Ovens)	30	7
Pita bread, white	30	10
Corn tortilla	50	12
Wheat tortilla	50	8

BEVERAGES

Coca Cola®, average	250	15
Fanta®, orange soft drink	250	23
Lucozade®, original (sparkling glucose drink)	250	40
Apple juice, unsweetened, average	250	12
Cranberry juice cocktail (Ocean Spray®)	250	24
Grapefruit juice, unsweetened	250	11
Orange juice, average	250	13
Tomato juice, canned	250	4

BREAKFAST CEREALS AND RELATED PRODUCTS

All-Bran™, average	30	4
Coco Pops™, average	30	20
Cornflakes™, average	30	21
Cream of Wheat™ (Nabisco)	250	17
Cream of Wheat™, Instant (Nabisco)	250	22
Grapenuts™, average	30	15
Muesli, average	30	16
Oatmeal, average	250	13
Instant oatmeal, average	250	17
Puffed wheat, average	30	16
Raisin Bran™ (Kellogg's)	30	12
Special K™ (Kellogg's)	30	14

GRAINS

Pearled barley, average	150	11
Sweet corn on the cob, average	150	17
Couscous, average	150	23
White rice, average	150	23
Quick cooking white basmati	150	23
Brown rice, average	150	18
White rice, converted (Uncle Ben's®)	150	14
Whole wheat kernels,	50	14

average		
Bulgur, average	150	12
COOKIES AND CRACKERS		
Graham crackers	25	14
Vanilla wafers	25	14
Shortbread	25	10
Rice cakes, average	25	17
Rye crisps, average	25	11
Soda crackers	25	12
DAIRY PRODUCTS AND ALTERNATIVES		
Ice cream, regular	50	8
Ice cream, premium	50	4
Milk, full fat	250	3
Milk, skim	250	4
Reduced-fat yogurt with fruit, average	200	7
FRUITS		
Apple, average	120	6
Banana, ripe	120	13
Dates, dried	60	42
Grapefruit	120	3
Grapes, average	120	8
Orange, average	120	5

Peach, average	120	5
Peach, canned in light syrup	120	9
Pear, average	120	4
Pear, canned in pear juice	120	5
Prunes, pitted	60	10
Raisins	60	28
Watermelon	120	4
BEANS AND NUTS		
Baked beans, average	150	7
Black-eyed peas, average	150	13
Black beans	150	7
Chickpeas, average	150	8
Chickpeas, canned in brine	150	9
Navy beans, average	150	12
Kidney beans, average	150	7
Lentils, average	150	5
Soy beans, average	150	1
Cashews, salted	50	3
Peanuts, average	50	1
PASTA and NOODLES		
Fettuccini, average	180	18
Macaroni, average	180	23
Macaroni and Cheese (Kraft)	180	32

Spaghetti, white, boiled 5 min, average	180	18
Spaghetti, white, boiled 20 min, average	180	27
Spaghetti, whole meal, boiled, average	180	16
SNACK FOODS		
Corn chips, plain, salted, average	50	17
Fruit Roll-Ups®	30	24
M & M's®, peanut	30	6
Microwave popcorn, plain, average	20	8
Potato chips, average	50	11
Pretzels, oven-baked	30	16
Snickers Bar®	60	19
VEGETABLES		
Green peas, average	80	3
Carrots, average	80	3
Parsnips	80	12
Baked russet potato, average	150	26
Boiled white potato, average	150	14
Instant mashed potato, average	150	17
Sweet potato, average	150	17

Yam, average	150	13
MISCELLANEOUS		
Hummus (chickpea salad dip)	30	0
Chicken nuggets, frozen, reheated in microwave oven 5 min.	100	7
Pizza, plain baked dough, served with parmesan cheese and tomato sauce	100	22
Pizza, Super Supreme (Pizza Hut)	100	9
Honey, average	25	10

---

[8] http://www.health.harvard.edu/newsweek/Glycemic_index_and_glycemic_load_for_1 00_foods.htm. "International tables of glycemic index and glycemic load values: 2002," by Kaye Foster-Powell, Susanna H.A. Holt, and Janette C. Brand-Miller in the July 2002 *American Journal of Clinical Nutrition*, Vol. 62, pages 5–56.

Body Mass Index (BMI)

Body Mass Index is the preferred method of measuring obesity for the majority of physicians and obesity researchers. The actual calculation of body mass index is performed by dividing the weight of a person in kilograms by their height in meters, squared (kg/m^2). In general, a healthy BMI would be between 19 and 25.

The World Health Organization uses a classification system using the BMI to define the terms *"overweight"* and *"obesity."*

- A BMI of 25 to 29.99 is defined as a **"Pre-obese."**
- A BMI of 30 to 34.99 is defined as **"Obese class I."**
- A BMI of 35 to 39.99 is defined as **"Obese class II."**
- A BMI equal to or greater than 40.00 is defined as **"Obese class III."**[9]

In general, it is widely accepted that people with their fat concentrated in their middle are at greater health risk than those that have their fat concentrated in other areas of their body.

Problems associated with BMI include the disagreement as to where the actual cutoff for each

---

[9] http://www.medicinenet.com/obesity_weight_loss/page3.htm#toci

category should be as well as the fact that it does not take into account the actual amount or the percentage of body fat.

The "Set Point" Theory

The Set Point Theory was developed when it was determined that each person has a unique established weight that their body tries to maintain. This theory states that as caloric intake rises and falls the body adjusts its metabolic rate to maintain its *"fat-to-muscle ratio."*

Research conducted at Rockefeller University showed that when a person gained weight their metabolic rate would increase in an attempt to return the body to its *"set point"* weight. Conversely when a person lost weight their metabolic rate would decrease in an attempt to return the body to its higher weight. This resistance to deviating from the "set point" weight is why many researchers believe diets don't work. The set point appears to be associated with how sensitive the fat cells are to insulin.

We will outline how to beat this resistance in future chapters so you can lose weight anyway and not get stuck in a rut like all those people unfamiliar with the Set Point Theory.

The "Fat Cell" Theory

This theory claims that fat cells are formed either during childhood or in early adolescence around puberty. This theory claims also that a child that consumes large amounts of fat can actually increase their number of fat cells. This is referred to *"hyperplastic obesity."*

This theory also claims that an adult will maintain the same number of fat cells and merely change the size of individual fat cells by changing their caloric intake and percentage of fat in their diet. If their caloric intake is increasing and the percentage of fat they consume is increasing they will most likely experience what is called *"hypertrophic obesity."*

While hyperplastic obesity is said to be rare, the statistics released by the CDC in 1999 stated that obesity in children and adolescents has more than doubled in the last two decades.[10]

The bottom line is that the majority of overweight people are of the hypertrophic obesity type. This means that you have not grown additional fat cells you just filled up the ones you already had. We are going to show you how to empty them as you progress toward the new thin and healthy you.

It has been shown in research released since this theory was published that adults can increase the number of fat cells as well as increase the size of their fat cells. This increase in the number of fat cells,

---

[10] http://www.cdc.gov/nchs/nhanes.htm http://www.faqs.org/nutrition/Met-Obe/National-Health-and-Nutrition-Examination-Survey-NHANES.html

called *hyperplasia,* generally occurs in specific situations such as during pregnancy, during late childhood and early puberty and in situations where large amounts of weight have been gained in a relatively short period of time.

Remember, your body uses carbohydrates for energy if the body needs energy. If it doesn't, the body stores the carbohydrates as fat. So don't eat a peanut butter and jelly sandwich and a bowl of processed cereal and sit on the couch for 3 or 4 hours if you want to lose your excess weight.

Diet-Induced Thermogenesis

Diet-induced *thermogenesis* is simply a measure of how much of the food intake is converted immediately to heat. Thin people have a higher percentage of their food being immediately converted to heat and therefore maintain a thinner build. Overweight and obese people experience a much lower percentage of this diet-induced thermogenesis and therefore convert less of their food intake immediately to heat. It is thought that a major factor for the lower level of diet-induced thermogenesis in overweight and obese people is due to insulin resistance or insensitivity. As mentioned earlier, this is often a result of the food choices being made.

The Physiological Process of Converting Fat to Energy

Fat is stored inside the fat cell, or *adipocyte*, in the form of *triaglycerol*. When energy is low, the fat cell is stimulated to release the triaglycerol in the form of free fatty acids or FFAs. The triaglycerol is split in a process known as hydrolysis into glycerol and 3 fatty acids. The enzyme, or catalyst, for this reaction is *Hormone Sensitive Lipase* or *HSL*. These FFAs are then transported through the bloodstream to the tissues needing the energy. These FFAs are then helped into the mitochondria of the cells of these tissues by an enzyme, *lipoprotein lipase (LPL)*. Once inside the mitochondria, the FFAs can be used for energy.

Remember that the adipocyte or fat cell is losing its contents in the form of glycerol and free fatty acids. If it is emptying its contents then it must be getting smaller and if your fat cells are getting smaller you must be losing weight and getting thinner.

A healthy adult with normal body composition has between 25 and 30 billion fat cells where an infant may only have 5 to 6 billion. The average weight of an adult fat cell is 0.6 micrograms (a microgram is one millionth of a gram or 1/1,000,000 gram). A pound of fat contains approximately 3500 calories. To lose a pound of fat each week you need to burn 3500 additional calories or eat 3500 less calories each week. This equates to 500 calories on a daily basis. Don't worry we are not going to start religiously counting calories. The book is called, *"Lose Weight Without Dieting"* and counting calories is dieting. Suffice it to say that you need to become familiar with foods and their total calories, their glycemic index and their glycemic load. This will simply help you to make better food choices in the future and lose the weight you want to lose and keep it off by limiting the amount of times you cheat and eat the wrong foods. Everything in life is a trade-off. If you get something for nothing that is generally what it's worth also.

Chapter 4: The Psychology of Weight Loss

In order to lose weight you must be convinced that you can do it. If you don't think you can then you're right, you cannot. If you have been on so many diets and had so many failures that you just cannot get the right mindset, see if some of the information in this chapter will help get you on track mentally.

Tony Robbins in his book, *"Awaken the Giant Within"* talks about using questions you ask yourself. The important aspect of asking these questions is, of course, to ask the right questions. I'll let him explain:

"Questions are undeniably a magic tool that allows the genie in our minds to meet our wishes, they are the wake-up call to our giant capacities. They allow us to achieve our desires if only we present them in the form of a specific and well-thought-out request. A genuine quality of life comes from consistent, quality questions. Remember, your brain, like the genie, will give you whatever you ask of it. So be careful what you ask for – whatever you look for you'll find. So with all this power between our ears, why aren't more people happy, healthy, wealthy, and wise? Why are so many frustrated, feeling like there are no answers in their lives? One answer is that when they ask questions, they lack the certainty that causes the answers to come to them, and most importantly, they fail to consciously ask empowering questions of themselves. They run roughshod over this critical process with no forethought or sensitivity to the

power they are abusing or failing to ignite by their lack of faith."[11]

Then he goes on to apply this concept of questioning yourself to the process of weight loss.

"A classic example of this is a person who wants to lose weight and can't. It's not that they cant: it's that their present plan of evaluating what to eat is not supporting them. They ask questions like 'What would make me feel most full?' and 'What is the sweetest, richest food I can get away with?' This leads them to select foods filled with fat and sugar – a guarantee of more unhappiness. What if instead they asked questions like 'What would really nourish me?' 'What's something light that I can eat that would give me energy?' or 'Will this cleanse or clog me?' Better yet, they could ask, 'If I eat this, what will I have to give up in order to still achieve my goals? What's the ultimate price I'll pay if I don't stop this indulgence now?' By asking questions like this, they'll associate pain to overeating, and their behavior will change immediately.

To change your life for the better, you must change your habitual questions. Remember, the patterns of questions you consistently ask will create either enervation or enjoyment, indignation or inspiration, misery or magic. Ask the questions that

---

[11] Anthony Robbins, *Awaken the Giant Within* (New York: Simon & Schuster, 1991), p. 185.

will uplift your spirit and push you along the path of human excellence."[12]

If you have never read any of Tony Robbins books I strongly recommend you start. They are not only entertaining to read, they will help you in ways you never dreamed possible!

Tony states that every decision we make, all of your neurological patterns, have been designed to get you out of pain and into pleasure. So the pain of being overweight must be overpowered by the pleasure of getting that excess weight off. This will allow you to gain the self-esteem you deserve and need for success at anything whether it is weight loss or quitting smoking.

You are going to need to consciously choose the patterns that will replace your overeating to ensure you do not replace one bad habit with another. You must interrupt the connection between overeating and pleasure and replace it with some positive behavior. Don't allow your brain to decide what the new pattern will be! Choose it consciously!

Maybe the reason that you have tried other diets and failed is because you failed to replace the old neural pathway of overeating with a new one. Maybe the triggers that cause you to overeat are still in place and external pressures like health issues or a spouse that is turned off by your excess weight are not enough for you to make lasting changes. You need to focus on the internal reasons for you to lose

---

[12] Robbins, *Awaken the Giant Within*, 186.

weight and replace those negative patterns, whatever they are, with positive ones that will assist you in achieving your goals once and for all! If you do not replace these negative patterns with new positive ones, it is unlikely that external pressure will result in the long-term changes you desire.

Your mind is a very powerful tool but most people fail to use it effectively to get what they really want in life. Imagine your overeating and all the negative it has created in your life. Visualize each time something negative happened because of your overeating or your present state of being overweight. Now, imagine how wonderful things will be when you lose the weight. Imagine how differently people will react to you. Imagine all the positive things that will happen when you finally get that weight off and are able to keep it off!

Run this positive visualization over and over in your mind. It may sound a little crazy but if it works so what. Maybe it is crazy, big deal! I assure you it does work! In your visualizations imagine how losing the excess weight you desire will move you from the painful experience of being overweight to the pleasurable experience of not having any of the excess weight. Do not fail to do these visualizations. Failing to do these visualizations will ensure that it is only a matter of time until you are back overeating, once again seeking pleasure from the wrong source.

Small achievements deserve rewards. Always reward yourself when you first begin to break the pattern of overeating. Maybe when you first eat a meal without the usual piece of bread or you finish a meal and don't have dessert. Naturally you will want to reward yourself with something other than more food. Remember you are breaking that pattern.

You might reward yourself by just saying to yourself,

"Good job! You're on your way!"

These rewards will cause your brain to associate these changes with pleasure. Don't try to reward yourself with things that are not really rewards. Your brain will not associate pleasure to them if you do. Don't replace dessert with celery unless you really like celery. Let's face it, if you really liked celery you wouldn't be reading this book and wanting to lose weight. The reward must be a true reward but not food.

Tony Robbins states in <u>Awaken the Giant Within</u> that,

"All patterns are the result of reinforcement; specifically, the key to creating consistency in our emotions and behaviors is conditioning."[13]

He also states in his, *"Law of Reinforcement"* that,

"Any pattern of emotion or behavior that is continually reinforced will become an automatic and

---

[13] Robbins, *Awaken the Giant Within*, 139.

conditioned response. Anything we fail to reinforce will eventually dissipate."[14]

Make sure to remember these principles laid out by Mr. Robbins. I strongly recommend buying one or more of his books. It will make a difference in your success.

I have dessert three times a year; Once at Christmas, once at Thanksgiving and once on my birthday. I feel nauseous after each time and for that reason I can easily go the rest of the year without dessert. The negative feeling I get after I eat these sugary, empty calories is enough to prevent me from wanting to have this kind of food the rest of the year. When I am offered a piece of cake or pie I can never answer immediately. In the old days I would have always said yes whether I was hungry or not. That didn't matter I was absolutely not going to miss out on a piece of cake. Now I think for about two seconds, remember how I feel after I eat that crap and then politely say, "No Thanks."

---

[14] Robbins, *Awaken the Giant Within*, 139.

Setting Goals

Everyone is familiar with setting goals and realizes that many of the exercises designed to help you set and achieve your goals don't work unless you have some strong inner determination to make the change. You need to think of the one primary reason you want to lose weight. This may be because someone wouldn't go out with you because of your weight or because you didn't have the confidence to apply for a particular job because of your size. It doesn't matter what it is that is motivating you. Simply stated, if you have a really strong desire to lose the excess weight you will have an easier time with the whole process. You need focus and determination to make these positive changes in your life.

Your goals also need to be concrete and specific otherwise it is like going into a travel agent and telling them you would like a plane ticket. When they ask you where you want to go you say, "Someplace nice." Guess what? They're going to think you're crazy. This however, is no crazier than expecting to get somewhere you have not precisely laid out and specifically described.

Write down your goals and read them every day without fail. Read them at least once in the morning and once in the evening. At the beginning you should read them 5 to 10 times every day to really get the mental and emotional ball rolling. You need to read them multiple times each day until they are permanently ingrained in your mind.

Meditation and or Yoga are also useful tools when making global changes to your life. They will help you have more focus and more inner control of your minute by minute decisions which, over time, will lead you to your desired outcome, a thinner healthier you. There are many good tools online that can teach you meditation techniques and Yoga positions.

Always remember, your feelings come from your thoughts and you control your thoughts. So, in essence, you control your feelings. Don't forget this simple point!

Chapter 5: The New Menu

Well, you're finally here. The **New Menu** will outline the foods that you will be eating to lose the desired pounds along with the foods to avoid to expedite the weight loss. The following pages will incorporate many of the things you have learned in previous chapters concerning the storage and use of fat for energy, the reasons why most diets fail and the various theories on weight loss.

Needed Items

The only items you will need are a steamer or steaming tray to set into a saucepan, a large bowl to store lettuce and some small bowls for vegetables. Besides that, all you will need is a knife to cut up vegetables, a carrot peeler and a cutting board. The main thing you will need is, of course, your willingness to give this **New Menu** a chance to work. Make sure to give it a month and document the changes you notice. That is, changes in your mood, your mental clarity, your energy levels and, of course, your weight.

By all means, take a picture before you start. That before picture will be a motivator like you would not believe when you hit a plateau or decide to give up because the diet isn't working anymore. When this happens simply take out the "Before" picture and look at it while you look at yourself in the mirror. You will notice the positive changes you have made and you will be right back on track losing the rest of the weight you want to lose.

Eliminate These Foods From Your New Menu

Even more important than the list of foods you should eat is the list of foods you should not eat. As an overweight person determined to lose the excess weight, you will need to absolutely eliminate certain foods completely at the beginning of this process and most of the time after that for the rest of your life if you wish to keep the weight off. Do not despair. I switched to this new menu and have never looked back. Sure I get hungry for the "other" foods and occasionally I partake but when I do I notice the next day I have what feels like the equivalent of a hangover for a drinker.

Milk and other dairy products are the bad guys when it comes to mucus production. It is difficult for some people to eliminate milk from their diet. If this is the case with you try some natural organic milk or almond milk from the health food store.

Natural organic milk can be bought at most grocery stores and almost all health food stores. Keep in mind that this milk has no antibiotics and no steroids. In other words, the cows that supplied the milk were not given steroids or antibiotics. Steroids cause the cow to produce more milk and therefore it can be produced cheaper. Similarly, natural organic milk without the antibiotics and steroids is more expensive.

Inflammation has been the focus of many new research studies and new findings are being uncovered every day but suffice it to say that inflammation is generally a negative response to some trauma. The trauma can be a wood splinter stuck in your finger or maybe even a response to a large refined sugar intake.

For these first three months you need to eliminate all sugars and sugary foods like cake, candy, pie, pudding, sweet tea, soda and even fruit as mentioned earlier. The only fruit you should eat for the first three months is green apples. In the menus I outline in coming pages you will notice various fruits such as blueberries and pineapple. Try to avoid even these at the beginning. After you begin to lose the desired weight you can start adding these in as a treat.

In addition, you need to eliminate the foods that convert to sugar rapidly in the body. These include bread, potatoes, pasta, rice and cereal or any processed grain product for that matter. Limit your grain intake to one or two servings per day after the first month and eliminate them completely for the first month.

When you do eat grains in the form of cereal or bread get the whole grain variety. The less processed the better. Many cereal and bread companies make exorbitant claims about how natural their product is but I strongly recommend that you get these products from a health food store to insure you are truly getting unprocessed grain products. Processed grain products will prevent you from losing much of the weight you would otherwise lose because they convert to sugar very rapidly since they are heavily processed.

As a general rule, if there is a picture of the food on the box, it is almost always very processed. The problem with processed foods is twofold. First of all, the nutrients have been processed out of the food and very little nutritional value remains. Secondly, chemicals are generally added to preserve the food almost indefinitely. These chemicals are dangerous to your health even in small amounts.

Many people confuse water retention and the resultant swelling or edema with inflammation. Excess water retention is generally a result of too much sodium in the diet but there are numerous other reasons that can cause water retention. This is covered more in the next section. If you are retaining water you should see a doctor. If the water retention is not severe you may try reducing your salt intake or replacing the sodium chloride (table salt) with potassium chloride (no salt).

Later, when you are through your first three months with the new menu you can begin to add a banana once or twice a week. Bananas are rich in potassium which replaces sodium as a positive ion in your body but does not cause water retention. If you do not want the calories and sugar that bananas contain you may wish to get some potassium bicarbonate capsules online or from your local health food store. I have been using these capsules for about a year. See the next chapter and Appendix A. I used to purchase these capsules from Naturamart but have been told that they are not selling them anymore.

After the initial couple of weeks you should start to see and feel some real improvements happening. Not just changes, noticeable improvements that you can see and feel.

We are all familiar with the low carb diets however it is not all carbohydrates we need to eliminate if we want to lose weight. We need only remove the simple carbs from our diet to produce the desired result.

The other carbohydrates, the complex carbs, should still be eaten and will therefore be included in the New Menu. Specifically, you should eliminate all breads and other grains. This means no cereal in the morning and no sandwiches at lunch. It is difficult at first to eliminate these foods as they are generally so much a part of our normal American diet. You may have to get a little creative to avoid these foods but your health and weight loss depend on it. This is one reason obesity is such a problem in our society. Almost everybody eats these foods in excess, most of us do not get enough exercise to burn up the extra energy so it is stored as fat and we end up a fat, obese country. Eliminating these foods for a time will make the difference between successful weight loss and frustrating weight fluctuations.

Grains are not the only carbohydrates you need to eliminate. Others include potatoes, rice, oatmeal, all fruit except for green apples. This will eliminate all of the foods that convert to sugar rapidly and cause you to gain weight and keep it on. Eliminate these foods and you will notice a difference in the way you feel almost immediately.

I said earlier to not throw these foods out keep them in the house to use during the transition period because it is hard to eliminate them from your diet. As you begin eating the right foods, begin eating less and less of the undesirable foods I mentioned above until they are gone from the cupboards and refrigerator. This usually takes a week or so. Do not continue to buy these foods until the desired weight has been lost. Sometimes a fleeting moment of weakness can be overcome by simply not buying the fattening food at all so eating it is not an option, it's not in the house.

In addition to the above foods you need to eliminate all sodas, candy, cake, ice cream, pie and anything else that has sugar in it.

I do not recommend that you use artificial sweeteners either. Studies have shown that people who use artificial sweeteners increase their affinity for sweets by using these artificial sweeteners containing aspartame. By increasing their affinity for sweets they increase their desire for sweets making it even more difficult to avoid eating them.

Keep in mind that every one of the previous artificial sweeteners has turned out to cause major health risks all the way back to cyclamates and saccharine in the 60s, 70s and 80s. Both of these previous artificial sweeteners were shown to cause cancer in laboratory rats and were taken off the market.

It has been shown that if aspartame is exposed to extreme temperatures it degrades down to a methyl alcohol compound which can cause serious health problems. My recommendation, don't use artificial sweeteners. Get used to the taste of things without adding sugar or sweetener. I drank coffee with cream and sugar for many years. Switching to coffee with cream only was like pulling teeth but I did it. I still don't like it as much but so what. It is much better to not have the sweets and I congratulate myself every morning for not having sugar or honey in my coffee. The reality is that I don't even keep these items in the house at all.

After the desired weight is lost, you can decide to pick a sweet prize for yourself once every week or two or even just once a month. Just don't go back to the old ways and add all these fattening and potentially unhealthy foods back into your diet on a daily basis. You will notice after you lose the weight and you are just dying for some fattening food that you have missed so much that after you eat it you feel like crap. I don't mean psychologically I mean actually physically feeling ill from eating the fattening food that of course has very little food value. At this point your body is wanting and expecting healthy food not worthless refined crap.

My weakness was always ice cream. Down the street from my house is a home-made ice cream shop. The scoops are huge and the flavor is fantastic. I finally went down to have my double scoop and after I was finished I felt about half sick. The next day I felt a little weak and not quite up to par. The only thing it could have been was the ice cream. Sometimes it isn't until we get truly healthy that we realize how crappy those foods we thought we loved actually make us feel.

I noticed that with salads. I didn't really get hungry for salads but I started forcing myself to eat one each day. I would tear 3 leaves of Romaine lettuce up into a bowl. To that I would add tomatoes, zucchini squash, yellow squash, white onion, broccoli and maybe some spinach leaves. You can mix and match the vegetables you like in your salad. I always use romaine lettuce because 3 leaves has 100% of the Vitamin B Complex needed by an adult for the entire day.

After about two months of my *"one salad a day"* regimen I woke up one morning actually craving a salad. It scared the hell out of me! What about donuts? What happened to that craving? Was I turning into Jack LaLane? I knew he ate this healthy and liked it I just never truly thought that I would. You will be surprised how easily you will adapt if you will just give yourself the chance to do so.

Give yourself at least a month to change your cravings, get your body cleansed and let the healthy food take effect. For dressing you should use red wine vinegar, balsamic vinegar or apple cider vinegar and extra virgin olive oil mixed 50-50. It's very light and not fattening. To this add sea salt and pepper to taste. Extra virgin olive oil is cold pressed and is the highest grade. Virgin olive oil is heat pressed so the yield is higher making the oil slightly cheaper.

This may sound gross compared to a peanut butter and jelly with a chocolate milk but trust me, you will adapt and your cravings will change to the point where the peanut butter and jelly doesn't even sound good because you know how it is going to make you feel. You will begin to associate those sluggish feelings and the indigestion with the foods that cause them and by eliminating them you will lose the weight and be able to keep it off. By the same token you will begin to associate salads and fresh healthy foods with energetic, clear-headed vibrant feelings. Once this starts to happen you are on your way and believe me it will!

    The last food you need to eliminate is cheese. The only cheese that you can eat that will not cause weight gain is cottage cheese. I don't know about you but I can't stand cottage cheese. It doesn't seem like real cheese. I remember in wrestling when the coach told us he would tell us one kind of cheese we would be allowed to eat and he said cottage cheese. We argued that cottage cheese was not even real cheese and he had to pick an actual cheese like American or Monterey Jack or something like that. Anyway, no luck. Cottage cheese was it. If you like it you're in luck.

    Yogurt is allowed but only the plain variety. That is not the vanilla flavored but the plain, no sugar. You will have a chance to have plain yogurt with fresh pineapple, blueberries and raspberries when you learn about the New Desserts that accompany many of the recipes. You will be surprised at how tasty they are even with the plain yogurt. You will actually start liking the plain yogurt. I certainly did not like it at the beginning but actually look forward to pineapple and plain yogurt for dessert or some berries with the yogurt. It tastes better than cake and ice cream to me now and it will not give you the awful feeling after you eat it like cake and ice cream do.

Even if those foods don't do that to you now, they will when you get healthy. Once you get used to no indigestion you really notice it when it returns. By the same token, when you experience indigestion two or three times a day, you hardly notice it after years and years of repeating the same experience.

Another thing you need to watch is condiments and sauces. These always seem to be very high in calories, sugar, salt and preservatives. Any time you can eliminate condiments and sauces do so. Pick up a ketchup bottle and read the ingredients. Notice where sugar or high fructose corn syrup are on the list and how near the top they are. Look at all the synthetic dyes they are including in these sauces and condiments.

Eliminating these sauces and condiments can leave your food tasting rather bland. The solution is simple. Use marinades. The dry marinades require either oil, vinegar or water or some combination of the three. I always buy the extra virgin olive oil and balsamic vinegar in both red and white. I generally marinade meats at least one whole day but sometimes even for two or three.

I used to have a habit of frying fish once a week. I knew fried food was not good for me but I figured it was only once a week and it is fish after all. I mean it's not like I'm frying a Twinkie, right. After finding and beginning to use marinades I tried marinating fish. For those of you who are familiar with marinating fish this is probably not so earth shattering but when I first made baked fish that I had marinated overnight I was amazed. It tasted like I was eating in a gourmet restaurant. It was actually better than the fried fish I thought I would have such a hard time giving up. I do occasionally make the home-made tartar sauce. I know it's not good for me but I have it every now and then anyway. Remember, you can cheat once in a while.

Include These Foods in Your New Menu

Certainly if you are trying to lose weight, the healthier you can eat the better. Your body needs every bit of ammunition and support you can give it to lose weight and get healthy. This is especially true if you are losing weight. There is no doubt that fattening foods leave acidic and other toxic residues that must be eliminated from the body. The fresher the food is the better. One thing I realized over time was that sugar and any food that is converted to sugar rapidly by the body seemed to cause weight gain or at least prevent weight loss. Was sugar causing the inflammation?

Fungi eat sugar so it is important to eat foods that do not contain any sugar and cannot be converted to sugar rapidly by the body like simple carbohydrates. These would include any sweet foods such as cake, pie, pudding, candy, soda, jelly, processed peanut butter and cereal. Also included are the foods that convert to sugar in a few biochemical steps. These are the simple carbohydrates mentioned earlier such as pasta, bread, potatoes, rice and other grains. You do not need to eliminate these foods forever just long enough to see if this may be at least part of the problem. You will need to eliminate all grains while attacking this potentially fungal related problem which includes cereal, corn on the cob and popcorn.

Make sure and document the changes as you begin utilizing this new diet.

Keep in mind, grains are harvested across the Midwest in late summer. These are the hottest, most humid months of the year. Grains are harvested and stored in grain elevators where mold and other fungi thrive in late summer. Adding the grain to the elevator adds the missing ingredient, the food supply for the fungi.

Corn is notorious for being infected with Aspergillus, a fungi or more specifically a mold. It was stated in the October 2002 Journal of the American Medical Association (JAMA) that corn is frequently contaminated with Aspergillus.

Protein is extremely important for proper brain function and optimal health especially when losing weight. In general, stick to fresh protein sources such as beef, pork, chicken, fish and lamb. If you can find a natural or health foods store that sells these protein sources it is recommended you pay the extra money and buy your protein there. The protein sources sold in health food stores generally have not been contaminated with antibiotics and steroids like the protein you generally find at the grocery store.

The meat, especially the beef, purchased from these health food stores has been grass fed. The highest quality beef is the "grass finished" beef. Grass finished beef just means they did not feed the cow corn in the weeks preceding butchering. Corn is generally fed to cows for about 6 weeks prior to butchering. As we learned above corn is frequently contaminated with Aspergillus mold. Aspergillus produces a mycotoxin called, *Aflatoxin B1*, a known carcinogen that has been shown to cause colon cancer.

If you do not have a health food store nearby you might check your local grocery. Many of them now sell protein sources without the antibiotic and steroid contamination. These choices are more expensive than the usual beef, pork, chicken and fish the grocery sells. Eggs and milk can also be found that do not have the contamination and they too are more expensive since yields are diminished when the animal is not given the antibiotics and especially the steroids.

Besides the fresh, uncontaminated meat, you should include fresh vegetables. Fresh vegetables contain enzymes that are extremely beneficial to everyone but especially for someone losing weight. Cooking the vegetables destroys the enzymes.

According to Dr. Baroody, author of the book *Alkalize or Die*, you need to eat 70% - 80% of your vegetables raw, as in a salad, and steam the other 20% – 30%. Stay with these two food components (protein and vegetables) until the weight you are trying to lose is eliminated. That is, the protein rich beef, pork, chicken, fish and lamb and the raw and steamed vegetables. I was never able to achieve the 70% to 80% raw vegetables but hovered around 50-50 which was enough to make a considerable difference.

When choosing fish make sure it is not from a fish farm. These farms contaminate the meat in the same manner that farmers contaminate beef, pork, chicken and lamb with antibiotics and steroids.

With this new menu you will notice that your thinking will become clearer, you will sleep more soundly, your mood will be more consistent and you will be more even tempered. I personally noticed these benefits as I transitioned to this new menu.

It is very difficult to adapt immediately to this New Menu but your life and certainly your health may very well depend on it. Keep in mind that you can have as much of the steamed and raw vegetables and protein as you want.

I typically fried fish or chicken once a week or so. I wanted to get away from the unhealthy fried foods but I didn't know any other way to prepare fish that tasted good. If you just bake it the result is so bland. The solution I found was marinade. I began buying dry packets of marinade at the local discount grocery along with olive oil and balsamic vinegar. I recommend using either balsamic vinegar or apple cider vinegar.

One of the most difficult elements of this New Menu is that all the foods I like to snack on are prohibited so, to say the least, it took a major adjustment to get used to it for me.

One problem at the beginning was that I had all the foods that were not allowed on the New Menu already in the house and I didn't want to just throw them out and buy all new food.

I made the transition to the New Menu over a two week period so as not to shock my system and as a result I didn't have to waste the food we already had in the house. This New Menu included much healthier foods than I was used to eating so I was going to benefit personally.

You will need to come up with something to have for snacks. Powdered donuts and chocolate milk are not on the menu but fresh cut salads are, so I began to eat salads once or even twice a day.

If you have trouble eating raw vegetables because they are to hard then the easy solution is to eliminate the hard vegetables from the salads and put them in the steamer. This is exactly what I did with carrots. Carrots are so hard many people have trouble chewing them. Put the carrots in the steamer and use some of the softer vegetables in the salad like zucchini squash and tomatoes.

When steaming your vegetables use a steaming basket that fits in a pan. You put water in the pan below the basket. I usually put garlic on every vegetable I steam. I use crushed garlic from a jar. Garlic helps lower blood pressure and cholesterol and it makes everything taste better, at least I think it does.

Something most people don't know about carrots is that they contain a natural anti-fungal substance called *falcarinol*. Falcarinol actually prevents the carrot from being consumed by fungi while it is growing in the ground. Without falcarinol not one carrot would ever grow.

In my reading I found out that while iceberg lettuce is not bad for you it has almost no vitamins or nutrients. However, I also found that three leaves of Romaine lettuce contain 100% of the vitamin B complex recommended for the entire day.

Anytime you can obtain your vitamins naturally from fresh foods, do so. I immediately switched to the slightly bitter Romaine lettuce and have never looked back. Every little bit of positive you can throw into the daily regimen helps.

Keep in mind that eating healthy is not like taking a pill that makes you feel better in an hour or so. Don't forget that once the effect of a pill wears off you're right back where you started. Eating healthy actually heals and repairs the body from years of abuse but it doesn't do it overnight.

This abuse is apparent in all of us with the possible exception of Jack LaLane. I remember seeing Jack when he was about 80 years young and he commented,

"You wouldn't give your dog a cup of coffee and a donut every morning because it would kill him. So why are you doing that to yourself?"

Quite obviously, Jack LaLane is a very wise man. You will need to drink water instead of soda or sweetened tea or coffee. I don't even have any sugar in the house and I haven't for almost 4 years now. Don't get me wrong, I do cheat every now and then. If you need to cheat, do it and then get back to the menu. The closer you adhere to this New Menu the sooner you will begin to lose all the weight you want to lose and begin to get your life back. You will notice that the closer you adhere to this New Menu and the longer the periods between cheating, the better you begin to feel and the more weight you will lose.

It is a lot like lifting weights. You get a little stronger each week and over the period of six months to a year, you get much stronger and begin to fill out your shirts to the point of them even being tight. The increase in size has been so miniscule from your perspective that you are sure the dryer is suddenly shrinking your clothes. It isn't shrinking anyone else's clothes, just yours.

It truly makes no sense but you are so sure you have not increased your size that it just must be that dryer. Then you see someone you haven't seen for a while and they ask what you have been doing because you look stronger. You saw the improvements every day which were so miniscule you failed to notice the long term improvement.

Don't let this happen with your health improvements. This is why I said earlier to document the improvements as soon as you begin the New Menu. Look every day for these little improvements and write them down along with the date. When you are feeling a little down and feel like you are not improving read the entries for a pick-me-up. This convinces you subconsciously that you are improving and your outlook changes to that of optimism and hope. Believing you are going to get thin and are improving a little each day greatly increases your ability to respond to these positive steps you are now taking.

I know I've said it a few times already but I'll say it again, you need to keep a diary. Record how you feel two or three times a day. Note each milestone and hurdle you overcome. When you have a bad day go back and look at the diary and read one of the days that you felt good for a reminder. This helps get your mind back on track and focused on getting thin and healthy.

    I mentioned cheating earlier. Straying from the New Menu is a bad idea in the first three months.

The Menu Transition

The transition is difficult so don't give in. Stick to your guns at the beginning and it gets easier. Don't throw away the fattening food you have in your cabinets, eat it. While you are eating the old fattening food
also mix in the healthy food from the New Menu. This will help you transition to the new way of eating that is going to change your life for good!

Notice the way you feel after eating some of the remaining fattening foods. Notice the sluggish, bloated way you feel. Notice the indigestion you feel that you have been ignoring all these years.

I remember when I first went to a chiropractor and he cracked my back. He actually was able to eliminate a dull roar pain I had been dealing with for many years. It generally went unnoticed since it had been there for so long. Since it was not a sharp pain I was able to somewhat ignore the pain for many years. Upon receiving the adjustment the pain went away although temporary, it was eliminated and I felt a rush of energy, presumably the energy that was being consumed in dealing with the pain.

As you begin to eat healthy and as you begin to eliminate the fattening, unhealthy foods from your diet you will realize how sick you feel when you eat those fattening, unhealthy foods. A sick feeling you have probably been ignoring for many years just as I had ignored the back pain for so long.

Snacks

As I mentioned earlier, this new menu does not offer much in the way of snacks. One snack that I found that my mom really likes is fresh blueberries and plain, natural yogurt. I don't mean vanilla flavored yogurt, I mean the plain yogurt that almost tastes like sour cream. I made this quick snack for my mother and much to my surprise she loved it. I was taking care of my mother who had emphysema and actually began to reverse her condition with this New Menu. Certainly there were more steps involved but this was the first step in her recovery, the recovery that the doctors said was impossible. It is not. To read more about how I reversed my mom's emphysema pick up the book, *"How I Reversed My Mom's Emphysema."* It is available on our web site at http://www.OptimalHealthProtocols.com or on http://www.Amazon.com.

You need to wait until after the first 3 months are over to have this snack because the blueberries are not recommended in the early stages of your weight loss process. Even though they are natural fruits, they contain sugar and will provide food for fungi.

I also went to http://www.KnowtheCause.com and found out what Doug Kaufmann said about snacking. His *Phase I* diet is similar to the diet that I have outlined above including protein and vegetables and eliminating sugar and foods that convert to sugar rapidly. Doug Kaufmann has had many years of success with patients after starting them on this diet.

You can also replace the blueberries with pineapple chunks. Always buy the pineapple fresh and cut it up yourself. Do not buy the canned pineapple. Pineapple contains bromelain, a proteolytic enzyme.

We will cover the benefits of proteolytic enzymes later in this book. Suffice it to say for now that pineapple is good for you and is especially good for you to eat if you have any debilitating condition associated with inflammation.

A snack that I got to like was almonds. For some people almonds are too hard to chew. If this is true for you also, all you need to do is soak them overnight in some distilled or filtered water. If you don't have distilled or filtered water you can use tap but I recommend not using tap water for any consumption. You can eat almonds, cashews, walnuts and pecans. Stay away from peanuts. Believe it or not, the skin on the peanut and the shell are easily and commonly contaminated with fungi such as mold. Another type of nut to stay away from is pistachios. Here again the skin and the shell allow for fungal contamination.

Another standby for a snack is raw vegetables with a little dip. You can use ranch dressing for the dip and even though it is not really on the menu you won't consume that much of it with your vegetables. If carrots are too hard for you to chew raw, use zucchini and yellow squash cut into strips. This makes an excellent snack and can be prepared when you are cutting up vegetables for your salads.

What I always do for salads is I tear up three Romaine hearts and put the lettuce into a large covered bowl I bought just for this purpose. I then cut up each vegetable including tomatoes and put each in its own bowl. I just buy the throw away storage containers you can buy at the grocery. This way you can make a salad quickly and it seems fresh. If you cut everything up and put it all in the bowl it only lasts maybe two days. After that it is not too appetizing.

Salads make excellent snacks and are one of the healthiest foods you can eat so get to the point where you enjoy them. I heard somewhere that it takes 30 days to change a habit. Within 30 days of eating salads every day you will begin to crave the raw vegetables and truly desire your daily salad.

After utilizing this new menu for about six months I had the weirdest experience. I woke up one morning and was actually hungry for a salad at breakfast time. Not donuts and coffee but a salad, raw vegetables! This had never happened to me before! I'm talking never in my life! I mention it only to demonstrate to you that you can adapt to anything healthy if you give it 30 days.

Start on this new menu immediately! There is no time to waste. Everything you have done up to this point has got you to where you are now. It is time to change this instant! Make out your new grocery list and then go through it and cross off the foods that are not allowed on the new menu.

Tracking Your Progress

It is important to track your progress but be reasonable. Don't weigh yourself every hour or even every day. At the beginning, when you are going through the transition weigh yourself every morning before you eat or drink anything and record your weight. At night before you go to bed weigh yourself again. This will show you the fluctuations in your weight from morning to evening and from one day to the next. In other words, you may be eating most of your fattening foods on the weekends when you are at home and no one sees you doing it. I remember seeing a bumper sticker that read,

"What you eat in private shows in public!"

Yes it's very rude but also very true. Since actually losing weight and keeping it off requires a lifestyle change not just counting calories or grams of carbohydrates. It is a change in attitude and focus. It is changing the things that trigger you to eat too much and to eat the wrong things. These triggers must be eliminated and replaced with triggers that cause you to eat healthy things and do healthy things.
Maybe instead of watching a movie with a bowl of ice cream you could go for a walk around the neighborhood or start riding your bike. Some friends of mine began playing Frisbee golf. It is not a lot of exercise but it is exercise and it gets you out of the house where the food is and gets your mind on

something else other than hunger and all the foods you are hungry for but know now that you shouldn't eat.

Making Better Choices

Making better choices comes with time. As you learn new meals that you like that are on the New Menu and record them mentally, your list of options grows. At the beginning you feel like you are going to have a hard time getting through another day because you can't figure out what you can eat. You just need to hang in there. At the beginning it seems the things that you need to eliminate from your diet make up the majority of your diet. Certainly change is difficult. Changing your diet is one of the most difficult things to do so if you have some rough times at the beginning give yourself a chance to adapt and grow into this new way of eating. I have supplied a number of menu options in Appendix A at the back of the book to get you started.

Cheating

What can I say, cheating is the nemesis of dieting. It undermines all that you have worked for and can easily negate all the progress you have made from your efforts and sacrifices so don't let your cheating get out of hand. On the other hand don't expect to never eat any of the items that are on the "DO NOT EAT" list. I used to reserve one day a week that I could eat anything I wanted. I could have beer, eat pizza and ice cream. I would look forward to that day all week and when it would finally arrive I would indulge myself all day long. How wonderful! The only problem was that I would feel nauseous after eating all that junk. I started only wanting to do my "cheat day" once every two weeks because I just didn't feel like having that sick feeling where I didn't want to do anything but lay around. I eventually went to one day each month and I have pretty much stuck with that regimen.

Once a month gives me enough time to forget the sick feeling from the last cheat day so I want to do it again. I do quite often skip my cheat day because I just don't want to eat those foods and feel like crap.

You will have to come to your own resolve with this issue but be very mindful of how often you cheat. You won't want to reverse all of the positive changes you have made in your life just for some ice cream or a few pieces of pizza. It's just not worth it! You will see what I mean in a few months when you start planning and looking forward to your cheat days and then don't enjoy them so much once they arrive. It's a confusing time. It almost seems like you don't have anything to look forward to anymore. All the foods you were so looking forward to eating after you lost your desired weight make you half sick now when you eat them. It's the price you pay for getting healthy.

After that we began to cheat once or twice a month for one meal or snack. You will notice that when you cheat you feel like crap the next day so you begin to not want to cheat near as often. You start asking yourself, "Do I really want to feel like crap just so I can have some ice cream?" After a while the answer, almost always, is no.

Chapter 6: Supplements for Sustained Health

Alfalfa and Cleansing

Alfalfa is an excellent cleanser due to its high chlorophyll content. It helps to alkalize the body by neutralizing excess acid and contains many vitamins in their natural state. (A, B, D, E, and K). Alfalfa can be bought very inexpensively at Wal-Mart in large containers holding 300 tablets at 650 mg each. If you have problems swallowing the rough tablets, dissolve them in water or tomato juice. This is one supplement that I think is okay to get at a large department store like Wal-Mart or K-Mart. There is not much to alfalfa just cut up grass pressed into a pill with a little binder to hold it together.

It will definitely cleanse your colon out so be careful not to take too much especially at the beginning until you know how your body will react to it. This is one of the best nutrients for anyone to take whether you are ill or not. I still take 8 to 12 tablets every day. My heartburn and acid reflux disappeared completely within a week of taking the alfalfa. I had suffered with heartburn and acid reflux for over 20 years when I learned about alfalfa and began taking it daily.

One thing you may not have realized is that unhealthy food is not just unhealthy while it is being eaten and digested, it leaves residue in many of your organs. Cleansing is the only way to eliminate these poisonous residues from your organs and your body as a whole. There are many cleansers out there and only a few that truly do what they claim to do.

I strongly recommend that you find a quality cleanser to cleanse these organs for three important reasons. First, ridding your body of the toxins that clog up your organs and prevent their efficient functioning is imperative for achieving optimal health. Second, cleansing your colon will cause weight loss by simply ridding your body of these rancid accumulations. Third, as you begin to eat healthy you will notice that instead of feeling tired after a meal you will be energized because you will be absorbing nutrient-rich foods. You cannot absorb these nutrient-rich foods if your colon is clogged up with accumulated garbage resulting from eating the wrong foods for many years.

I have found alfalfa to be an excellent cleanser that will continually cleanse your colon, your kidneys and your liver. It also moves you toward a more alkaline existence. This alkalinity will also help if you have heartburn or acid reflux. I had it for many years and used to take one roll of Tums™ every day. Since starting with alfalfa over 4 years ago I have not had heartburn or taken even one Tums™.

You may have experience cleansing your organs and have a product that you like and are accustomed to using. If this is the case remember to cleanse three or four times a year, roughly every 3 or 4 months. I prefer the alfalfa because it contains vitamins in their natural state, it contains chlorophyll which aids in cleansing and reducing acidity and it is very inexpensive. It is one of the few supplements I recommend buying from Wal-Mart. It is less than $4 for 300 650 mg tablets.

Vitamins and Minerals

It is imperative that you take a quality vitamin and mineral supplement whether you are ill or not. I believe that Primal Nutrition has the premier solution. Their Master Formula has the highest quality and most complete vitamin, mineral, antioxidant and phytonutrient supplement I have ever found. It is not cheap but it is well worth the price. It costs over $100 per month so it figures out to be $25 to $27 per week.

Besides vitamins and minerals, the Master Formula also contains antioxidants and phytonutrients that will help you regain your health. You will need a few other supplements but this will take care of the majority of your general supplement needs.

For example, most vitamin tablets contain Vitamin E as *tocopherol*. The Master Formula has the complete Vitamin E with all nine vitamin E's including 5 *tocopherols*. The Master Formula is also extremely fresh and is sent directly from their production facility to your door. No storing in hot warehouses for months on end as it is with many of the other vitamins on the market.

Make sure you get high quality vitamins. If you cannot afford the Master Formula find another high quality vitamin supplement to meet these needs. The Master Formula can be purchased from Primal Nutrition at *http://www.PrimalNutrition.com*.

Mark Sisson is the president of Primal Nutrition. Mark is a former Olympic triathalete and really did his homework when developing this formulation.

If you cannot afford The Master Formula you may wish to purchase some less expensive vitamins and minerals. Go to a health food store so you can make sure to get high quality, fresh vitamins.

Vitamins and minerals are enzymes and co-enzymes in biochemical reactions that occur during digestion. Without them your food will not break down as much as it would have with them. This means that maybe digestion does not occur completely which may cause indigestion. Also, since you are not breaking down your food completely you are missing out on some nutrients from your food that you would have otherwise absorbed. So get the most out of your food by always taking a vitamin and mineral tablet with every meal.

If you have invested in a premium vitamin and mineral product such as The Master Formula from Primal Nutrition you are ahead of the game.

Probiotics

Probiotics are probably one of, if not the most important supplement for anyone wishing to regain their health. Probiotics, as mentioned earlier in this book, are your first line of defense against fungi. Nearly everyone has *Candida albicans*. It's when this fungi or yeast is allowed to proliferate out of control for long periods of time that it seems to cause problems. If you have taken antibiotics then most likely your probiotics are nonexistent and your body will have a difficult time fighting off this otherwise innocuous fungi.

I found that Dr. Ohirra's Probiotics were enteric coated which allowed it to survive the stomach acid and break apart when it reached the small intestine. While more expensive than the other brands, Dr. Ohirra's seemed to replenish the probiotics lost to antibiotics and helped to restore my mother's health along with the new Menu and other supplements. There are also some very helpful medications we will cover later in this book.

There are other probiotics on the market. Even yogurt contains *Lactobacillus acidophilus*, a common probiotic. Some yogurts contain other species from the *Lactobacillus* genus such as *Lactobacillus regularum*. There is probably nothing wrong with other brands however, I had good luck with Dr. Ohirra's and I continue to use them even today.

I had been diagnosed with Attention Deficit Disorder (ADD) two decades earlier. I had neglected to take medications for the problem and forced myself to overcome it one day at a time. Sometimes that was an impossible task. The new Menu and Dr. Ohirra's Probiotics have now reversed my ADD. I didn't think that was possible until I began to research a myriad of health issues and healthy treatments for common yet debilitating ailments.

 ADD is certainly not a serious, life threatening disorder like emphysema, diabetes or cancer. I only mention it here because I thought you might find it interesting to hear the New Menu and probiotics may help with other disorders. Dr. Fred Pescatore, an MD in New York City and author of, *"The Allergy and Asthma Cure"* swears by this new Menu and Dr. Ohirra's Probiotics. If you or someone you know has allergies or asthma, check out Dr. Pescatore's book.

Omega-3 Fatty Acids

There are numerous benefits to supplementing Omega-3 and Omega-6 fatty acids. Volumes have been written on their benefits. For brevity sake, I have listed the main benefits of taking these supplements below. First of all, they are "essential." Essential in biochemistry simply means that your body does not produce it and you will need to supplement this nutrient either with your diet or by taking it as a supplement.

With many supplements you are better off taking a cheap supplement rather than not taking it at all. With the omegas this is not necessarily the case. Cheap omegas, often times, break down into free radicals that can actually damage your cells and cause them to age or even die.

I have used and can recommend either Nordic Naturals Omega-3 or Dr. Murray's Pharmaceutical Grade Omega-3 which are from, I believe, the New Factor company. Both will do the trick. I generally use the Nordic Naturals formula however, Dr. Murray's is nice because the pharmaceutical grade is twice the potency of the Nordic Naturals so it means you swallow half as many each day. Try to take at least 3 to 4 grams of Omega-3 each day.

The two primary omega-3 fatty acids are EPA (Eicosapentaenoic Acid) and DHA (Docosahexaenoic Acid). Both are key components for the health of both body and mind. GLA (Gamma Linolenic Acid) an important omega-6 fatty acid is also extremely important for optimal health. Listed below are some of the primary functions and benefits of these essential fatty acids.

EPA (Eicosapentaenoic Acid)

- Helps to maintain a healthy heart and circulatory system.
- Enhances joint flexibility and movement.
- Promotes healthy immune function.
- Supports healthy metabolism and body composition.
- Promotes balanced blood sugar levels.
- Supports the body's natural anti-inflammatory response.

DHA (Docosahexaenoic Acid)

- Supports learning and memory.
- Promotes positive mood and well-being.
- Supports and protects the brain, eyes and nervous and immune systems.
- Essential for the proper development of infants and children.
- Recommended by physicians for pregnant and lactating women.

GLA (Gamma Linolenic Acid)

- Nourishes hair and skin.
- Supports healthy joints.
- Enhances hormonal balance.
- Maintains normal body fat metabolism.
- Provides a "feel good" effect and improves moods.
- Promotes beneficial hormone-like cell messenger molecules that regulate swelling.

Dosages

Most countries recommend that adults consume at least 1 to 2 grams of the Omega-3 fats EPA and DHA, per day. Although there is yet to be an established daily value in the United States, the White House has advocated for the consumption of Omega-3 fatty acids, and the American Heart Association recommends EPA and DHA to individuals with heart disease.

Research into the importance of essential fatty acids (EFAs) began over 30 years ago. Today, there are thousands of scientific studies showing that EFAs play a critical role in human health.

The evidence is so convincing that health policy makers worldwide including, The American Heart Association, World Health Organization, and The British Nutrition Foundation have agreed that EFAs maintain health and prevent disease. International experts agree that adults require a minimum of 650 mg of the essential fatty acids, EPA and DHA, daily.

I personally take 3,000 to 4,000 mg of Omega-3 fatty acids every day. If you have trouble swallowing the capsules, Nordic Naturals also provides their Omega-3 formulation in liquid form as do some of the other quality omega-3 producers.

Absorption

Triglycerides contain a glycerol backbone, stabilizing the oil molecules in their natural form. But fish oils that are in the synthetic ethyl ester form are highly unstable, and rapidly break down during storage.

Additionally, when fish oils are digested they are converted into free fatty acids. After absorption through the epithelial cells, free fatty acids are immediately reassembled back into triglycerides by re-attaching to a glycerol backbone. If the glycerol backbone is missing (as they are with synthetic ethyl esters), and no other glycerol backbones are available, the oil cannot be converted back to triglyceride form. Fatty acids not converted to triglycerides pose an oxidation burden in the form of free radical formation.

Omega-3 fatty acids fall into two major categories: plant-derived (from flax seed, containing the shorter chain fatty acid, alpha-Linolenic, or ALA) and marine-derived (from fish oil, containing the longer chain fats, EPA and DHA). EPA and DHA are the fats that the body needs for health maintenance and enhancement.

While it was once thought that humans could convert the plant source (ALA) into EPA and DHA, research now shows that only about 5% of ALA converts to EPA, and that it may not convert to DHA at all. EPA and DHA from fish oil are the best and most efficient forms in which to consume Omega-3 fats.

Antioxidants and Phytonutrients

It is hard to read anything about healthy eating or reversing the aging process that doesn't include information about antioxidants. The antioxidant properties of Vitamins A, C, and E have been well documented and publicized. Although everyone seems to realize their importance, not many people understand how and why antioxidants work. You may have heard that they destroy "free radicals" which is true but what is a free radical? A free radical is a chemical compound that has an unpaired electron which causes it to be very unstable. This unpaired electron causes the molecule to have a charge which causes it to damage the cells and tissues of your body when it comes in contact with them.

Free radicals are created (initiation step) when these molecules are irradiated or when an incomplete reaction occurs in the body. Since these free radicals have an unpaired electron and a charge, they try to react with other molecules to neutralize this charge and become stable. These other molecules may be part of a cell wall, an important enzyme or even a DNA molecule. At any rate they cause damage when they react with different molecules in your body which can cause infection, disease or other debilitating conditions.

Antioxidants are substances whose function is to counteract the damaging effects of the physiological process of oxidation. Types of free radicals include the superoxide anion, the hydroxyl radical (OH^-), transition metals such as iron and copper, nitric acid, and ozone. The free radicals that contain oxygen are the most biologically important ones. They are referred to as reactive oxygen species or ROS and include the superoxide anion, the hydroxyl ion and molecules with oxygen that do not have an unpaired electron such as hydrogen peroxide.

There are actually two types of antioxidants. The first stops the chain reaction of one free radical stealing an electron and forming another free radical which in turn steals another electron and forms still another free radical and on and on and on until a termination step occurs. Examples of the antioxidants that stop this chain reaction are beta carotene, vitamin C and vitamin E. They are referred to "Chain-breaking" antioxidants.

The other type of antioxidants are "Preventive" antioxidants. They actually stop the initiation step of the free radical formation and prevent its creation. Examples of the preventive type of antioxidants are enzymes like *superoxide dismutase, catalase*, and *glutathione peroxidase.*

In addition to the antioxidants that have been mentioned above there are minerals that are necessary to make them work properly such as selenium, manganese and zinc. *CoEnzyme Q10* exhibits antioxidant properties and is important for energy production and protects the body from free radicals.

Below is a table that shows the recommended daily allowance and the upper level that you should not exceed when taking antioxidants.

Antioxidant Dosages

Antioxidant	RDA (adults)	Upper Level (adults)
Vitamin E	15 mg	1,070 mg natural vitamin E
Vitamin C	Women: 75 mg Men: 90 mg	2,000 mg
Beta-carotene	None	None
Selenium	55 mcg	400 mcg

What Foods Have These Antioxidants ?

Vitamin E foods containing vitamin E include but are not limited to leafy green vegetables, walnuts, almonds, seeds, olives and avocados.

Vitamin C citrus fruits (like oranges and grapefruit), broccoli, leafy green vegetables, tomatoes, peppers, cantaloupe, and strawberries.

Beta Carotene cantaloupe, mangoes, papaya, pumpkin, peppers, spinach, kale, squash, and apricots.

Selenium seafood, beef, pork, chicken, Brazil nuts, and whole wheat bread.

Phytonutrients

Some phytonutrients are currently being studied with a focus on their antioxidant properties and therefore their ability to reduce the potential for disease. They are listed below along with the foods that contain them.

Allyl sulfides	Onions, garlic, leeks, chives
Carotenoids (e.g., lycopene, lutein, zeaxanthin)	Tomatoes, carrots, watermelon, kale, spinach
Curcumin	Turmeric
Flavonoids (e.g., anthocyanins, resveratrol, quercitin, catechins)	Grapes, blueberries, strawberries, cherries, apples, grapefruit, cranberries, raspberries, blackberries
Glutathione	Green leafy vegetables
Indoles	Broccoli, cauliflower, cabbage, Brussels sprouts, bok choy

Isoflavones (e.g., genistein, daidzeins)	Legumes (peas, soybeans)
Isothiocyanates (e.g., sulforaphane)	Broccoli, cauliflower, cabbage, Brussels sprouts, bok choy
Lignans	Seeds (flax seeds, sunflower seeds)
Monoterpenes	Citrus fruit peels, cherries, nuts
Phytic acid	Whole grains, legumes
Phenols, polyphenols, phenolic compounds (e.g., ellagic acid, ferulic acid, tannins)	Grapes, blueberries, strawberries, cherries, grapefruit, cranberries, raspberries, blackberries, tea
Saponins	Beans, legumes

Nopal Cactus

Nopal Cactus acts like a sponge absorbing and expanding upon contact with the water and sugars in the stomach. The absorptive properties are temporary, allowing the slow release of the water and sugars back into the body, thereby helping to reduce sugar spiking immediately after a meal or drink. The high insoluble fiber content (cellulose and lignin) absorbs wastes in the intestines and bowels, pushing them along into and through the colon, making Nopal cactus an excellent cleanser.

The Nopal Cactus (*Opuntia strepacantha*) is a desert plant that survives intense heat and drought because of its ability to absorb and retain moisture in the mucilaginous fiber contained in its large flat spiny leaves. This insoluble fiber acts as a natural sponge holding the water, vitamins, minerals and essential amino acids in jelly-like mass which stores the cactus water and nutrients (which is called *"baba"* in Mexico) protects the cactus from sudden water loss, by slowly flowing from the leaf, similar to sap from a maple tree. Upon contact with the air, the baba is able to seal the flow of moisture from the leaf.

The Nopal Cactus is even available at many health food stores.

Seaweed

Seaweed is one of the primary sources of nutrition for ocean life. Seaweed is an excellent source of fiber, minerals, protein, and chlorophyll (10mg/100 grams), is rich in antioxidants and represents up to 10% of the diet in many Asian countries. Seaweed is an excellent cleanser, digestive aid, detoxification nutrient and source of calcium and iron.

Iodine is an important trace mineral found in seaweed. One serving of seaweed powder (10 grams) contains 0.12 mgs of iodine or 59% of the suggested daily value. For most people, iodine is an essential mineral helping to regulate the thyroid. However, persons with a thyroid condition should first consult with their health care professional to determine their limit of iodine consumption. Iodine has show to be a very important nutrient to consume in the event of exposure to high doses of radiation, interfering with the absorption of radioactive isotopes by the thyroid.

The seaweed can also be purchased from Seagate. I use many Seagate products because of their freshness and the company's attention to detail. The do not cut corners to increase profits. They deliver quality products consistently every time.

Fiber

Everyone is aware of the importance of fiber whether they know why it is important or not. It will promote the survival of your probiotics, the good bacteria in your small intestine by providing it with a food supply. Many of the good probiotics include in their formula a pre-biotic mixture to feed the bacteria until you ingest it and the enteric coating is removed. This will obviously enhance your immune system. Fiber can make you feel less hungry. Fiber can also assist in maintaining healthy blood glucose levels by slowing the absorption of sugars. It will also help cleanse your colon and assist with regularity and elimination of the toxins and fermented food residue lining your colon.

It is estimated that only about 10 percent of Americans get the recommended amount of fiber in their daily diet.[15]

The experts tell us that 32 grams per day of fiber is ideal for optimal health while most Americans get 10 to 15 grams daily. Those on low carbohydrate diets may only get 7 or 8 grams since the carbohydrates they are limiting contain the fiber they need to ensure optimal health.[16] Could this be the reason there is so much colon cancer in America?

Fiber comes in the soluble and insoluble varieties. Three common and easily found foods with considerable fiber are green beans, cauliflower and

---

[15] http://www.faqs.org/nutrition/Erg-Foo/Fiber.html
[16] http://www.faqs.org/nutrition/Ca-De/Carbohydrates.html

peas available at any grocery store in the country. You don't have to go to a specialty store or the local health food store to find them.

Psyllium is a very good source of soluble fiber that should be in your diet whether you are losing weight or not. Psyllium has been shown to lower cholesterol when accompanied by a diet low in saturated fats.

Potassium Bicarbonate

According to an article in the American Journal of Clinical Nutrition, the pre-agricultural diet included over 3 times as many bicarbonate producing foods than the current American diet.[17]

Americans average less than half the recommended daily intake of 4700 mg of potassium. Below is a partial list of some foods and their potassium content.

One sweet potato 694 mg
1 cup of tomato paste 664 mg
1 cup lima beans   484 mg
(but they are acidifying)
1 cup winter squash   448 mg
(but it is acidifying)
One banana   422 mg
1 cup cooked spinach 419 mg
1 medium cantaloupe 368 mg
1/2 cup lentils   365 mg
(but acidifying)
1/2 cup kidney beans   358 mg
(but acidifying)
One small apple   140 mg

Potassium, magnesium and calcium, the critical minerals for maintaining cell and blood health, are deficient in our diets.[18]

---

[17] American Journal of Clinical Nutrition, 2003, 76: 1308-1316

[18] POTASSIUM BICARBONATE ANTIDOTE TO DISEASE??, C. Norman Shealy, M.D., Ph.D., http://www.selfhealthsystems.com/archiveletter.php?id=240

Dietary potassium deficiency is a major contributor to hypertension as well as many diseases. Interestingly, potassium bicarbonate significantly reduces calcium excretion even in high protein diets. And there is evidence that potassium bicarbonate helps prevent osteoporosis through its calcium saving effect.

High protein diets, common in our society, are well known for their negative effect upon calcium. And interestingly, potassium bicarbonate also reduces nitrogen secretion as well as magnesium excretion. The combined benefits of potassium bicarbonate of enhancing calcium, magnesium and protein retention, while enhancing water excretion, are metabolically beneficial. Indeed, there is considerable evidence to suggest that potassium bicarbonate supplementation may well help prevent osteoporosis, reduce blood pressure, reduce weight and even improve adult onset diabetes. Theoretically, an increase in alkalinity might also reduce the risk of cancer.[19]

Most people are unaware that the adequate intake (AI) for potassium is 4,700 mg daily compared to the adequate intake for calcium is only 1200 mg. To provide a balance between acids and bases in the body it maintains alkaline reserves in the blood and tissues as well as other fluids in the body. Your bones also store additional alkaline reserves for use in neutralizing excessive acidic situations in the body. To read more about the necessity for all of us to

---

[19] European Journal of Nutrition, 2001, 40: 200-213.

alkalinize you may want to read, *Alkalize or Die* by Dr. Baroody.

Bone mineral reserves and matrix are compromised when all other alkalizing reserves are exhausted. This leads to the breakdown of bone structure and if it continues long-term it can, and probably will, lead to osteoporosis. So we see that it is probably our acidic diet that leads to osteoporosis. One more vote for green, leafy vegetables and their alkalizing effects along with the possible supplementation of potassium bicarbonate and alfalfa.

In research studies it has been shown that it is the bicarbonate that actually provides the alkalizing effects and the ultimate reversal of osteoporosis and its debilitating side-effects.

Fruits, vegetables, seeds and many spices contain large amounts of alkalizing potassium salts. The body converts these potassium salts to potassium bicarbonate. As we have already seen, the potassium bicarbonate is used by the body to neutralize metabolic acids. If you do not consume these potassium salts in your diet either from the food you eat or the supplements you take, minerals are robbed from your bones to neutralize the low grade metabolic acidosis.

Alkalizing Foods

Please note here that your diet should be 75% alkaline producing foods. Following is a short list of alkalizing foods.

Virtually all vegetables
Almost all fruits
Almonds
Millet
Tofu
Whey
Most seasonings, especially cinnamon, curry, ginger and herbs
Soured dairy products

Acidifying Foods

Note here that in an ideal situation only 25% of your diet should be acid producing foods.

Corn
Lentils
Olives
Winter squash
Blueberries
Cranberries
Currants
Plums
Prunes
All grains, flours and pastas, other than millet and chia
All beans and peas, including soy
Soy milk
Cheese
Eggs
Carbonated water
Ice cream and ice milk
Cashews
Peanuts
Pecans
Walnuts
Oils and fats, except olive oil
Canned fruits
All meats, including fish and fowl
Beer, liquor and wine
Soft Drinks
Coffee

Sugar
Mustard
Pepper
Carob
Vinegar
Aspirin and virtually all drugs, OTC as well as Rx
Herbicides
Pesticides
Tobacco
STRESS[20]

---

[20] Journal of the American Dietetics Association 1995;95:791-797

Kyolic Aged Garlic

A major research study in Canada revealed that 40% of the people taking an aspirin a day can actually increase their risk of stroke and heart attack. Three additional studies done in the U. S., Germany and Britain support these findings. Aspirin accelerates the breakdown of your joint cartilage. Aspirin can also cause gastrointestinal bleeding and over time can promote ulcers in your stomach and GI tract.

You might want to try aged garlic as an alternative and avoid these potentially life-threatening side-effects. A long-term study in the U. S. revealed that aged garlic extract actually lowered platelet aggregation and in turn, increased blood flow by 25%. Platelet aggregation is the propensity of platelets to stick together slowing blood flow. Aged garlic extract caused the platelets to not stick together due to the *methyl allyl trisulfate* and therefore improved blood flow.

In another study, aged garlic extract improved microcirculation or capillary blood flow and relaxed the smooth muscles of the arterial wall. Besides improving blood circulation and many other cardiovascular risk factors, it has also been shown to enhance immune function and protect your cells from oxidation and aging. Aged garlic extract has also been shown to detoxify your liver by quickly eliminating toxic chemicals.

Aged garlic extract has also been shown to improve your physical strength and reduces stress and fatigue as well as improving your memory function and enhancing nerve growth. Garlic is a natural antibiotic that does not eradicate your probiotics or "good bacteria" in your small intestine like prescription antibiotics do. Many fungal infections like yeast vaginitis, systemic candidiasis, and athlete's foot respond favorably to garlic; also certain viral infections like cold sores (fever blisters), some types of influenza, smallpox, and genital herpes.[21]

---

[21] http://www.healingwithnutrition.com/products/kyolicgarlic.htm/products/kyolicgarlic.htm

Supplements, Dosages & Frequency

Along with changing your diet to the one already outlined in the New Menu, you should also look into taking some very helpful supplements that have been outlined above. In this section we will cover which supplements, what dosages and how often you might want to take them.

At the beginning we were extremely cautious even though these were supplements bought at health food stores or online from health food companies. Most of these supplements are not exclusive to weight loss but are necessary for optimal health and therefore, apply here as well.

First of all, at each meal I recommend taking a vitamin and mineral tablet. Without them complete breakdown and utilization of the food you consume does not occur. I started with some cheap vitamins and graduated up to high quality, more expensive brands that were considerably more effective. The best vitamin, mineral, antioxidant, phytonutrient formula I have found is the Master Formula from Primal Nutrition. See Appendix 2 for ordering information.

Start with a quality vitamin and mineral formula from your local discount health food store. I always take one at each meal since these vitamins and minerals are enzymes and co-enzymes in biochemical reactions. They catalyze or "speed up" the reactions that may not otherwise occur prior to completing digestion. Essentially, you will get more benefit (utilization) from the food you are eating with vitamins and minerals.

Most of us have fungal infections. The way we get these fungal infections begins with antibiotics. Once we take antibiotics we kill the probiotics, the good bacteria. These probiotics are our first line of defense against *Candida albicans*, a common yeast and a member of the fungi family. The doctors may deny this fact but if you check their medical school curriculum you will find that, at least in most medical school curriculums the Mycology classes have been eliminated and replaced with additional drug classes. I recommend trying some of these anti-fungal supplements. If you experience a nauseous feeling in the first week or two on the New Menu you are probably experiencing what is called the *Herxheimer Reaction*. The *Herxheimer Reaction* is the *"die off"* of the fungus. The New Menu, along with getting you thin, is also designed to kill any fungal infection by removing its food supply. The New Menu takes away its food supply which is sugar and, of course, anything that converts to sugar rapidly.

The anti-fungal supplements should be cycled. That is, take one anti-fungal supplement one month and then change to a different anti-fungal supplement the next month and a different one again the third month. After this three month cycle you can repeat the anti-fungal supplements from the first month essentially starting the 3 month cycle over. Cycling the anti-fungal supplements prevents the fungi from adapting to the supplements which ultimately would render them ineffective.

If you are not sure if you have a fungal infection, you might want to take the Candida Self Test shown on the following pages. Dr. A. V. Constantini of the World Health Organization stated that,

"Fungal infections are the most overlooked medical problem in the world."

Dr. Constantini is a world renowned author and has written the Hope at Last series of books on breast cancer and prostate cancer. If you know anyone who is suffering from these cancers you might want to pick up a copy of these books.

Dr. Ohirra's 12 Plus Probiotics should be taken three in the morning and three in the evening for 10 days. This will use up one box. After that take two in the morning and two in the evening for 15 days and then go to one in the morning and one in the evening for the next two to three months to make sure the probiotics have repopulated your small intestines and are fully functional.

This is the regimen laid out by Cass Ingram, D.O., an osteopath and spokesman for Essential Formulas who market the Dr. Ohirra's 12 Plus Probiotics. You can find them on the internet at http://www.EssentialFormulas.com.

Now that you have implemented the New Menu and are taking your supplements religiously, it's time to take a look at other factors that will make a difference in your weight loss success.

The following pages contain the *Candida Self Test*. Make sure and spend some time to take the test and total your score. Look at what your score means in terms of the probability that you have a fungal infection involving *Candida albicans* or some other fungi.

Clinical Mycology textbooks state that these fungal infections are believed to be the underlying cause of many of the current debilitating diseases our society is suffering from. Could this be the reason your doctor prescribes medications to "manage" your disease and they don't seem to have any medications that actually "cure" disease?

Fungal Infection – SELF TEST

SECTION 1: HISTORY

1. Have you taken *tetracyclines* (*Sumycin®, Panmycin®, Vibramycin®, Minocen®*, etc.) or other antibiotics for acne for 1 month (or longer)?

    Enter 35 for Yes, 0 for No

2. Have you, at any time in your life, taken other *"broad spectrum"* antibiotics for respiratory, urinary or other infections (for 2 months or longer, or in shorter courses 4 or more times in a 1-year period)?

    Enter 35 for Yes, 0 for No

3. Have you taken a broad spectrum antibiotic drug — even a single course?

    Enter 6 for Yes, 0 for No

4. Have you, at any time in your life, been bothered by persistent *prostatis*, *vaginitis* or other problems affecting your reproductive organs?

    Enter 25 for Yes, 0 for No

5. Have you been pregnant? (enter only 1 answer)

    *2 or more times? Enter 5 for Yes, 0 for No
    *1 time? Enter 3 for Yes, 0 for No

6. Have you taken birth control pills? (enter only 1 answer)

   *For more than 2 years?
   Enter 15 for Yes, 0 for No

   *For 6 months to 2 years?
   Enter 8 for Yes, 0 for No

7. Have you taken prednisone, Decadron® or other cortisone-type drugs? (enter only 1 answer)

   *For more than 2 weeks?
   Enter 15 for Yes, 0 for No

   *For 2 weeks or less?
   Enter 6 for Yes, 0 for No

8. Does exposure to perfumes, insecticides, fabric shop odors or other chemicals provoke? (enter only 1 answer)

   *Moderate to severe symptoms?
   Enter 20 for Yes, 0 for No

   *Mild symptoms? Enter 5 for Yes, 0 for No

9. Are your symptoms worse on damp, muggy days or in moldy places?

   Enter 20 for Yes, 0 for No

10. Have you had athlete's foot, ring worm, *"jock itch"* or other chronic fungal infections of the skin or nails? Have such infections been, (enter only 1 answer)
    *Severe or persistent?

Enter 20 for Yes, 0 for No

*Mild to moderate?
Enter 10 for Yes, 0 for No

11. Do you crave sugar or sugar containing foods like desserts and candy?

    Enter 10 for Yes, 0 for No

12. Do you crave breads, rolls, muffins or any other grains or foods made from grains?

    Enter 10 for Yes, 0 for No

13. Do you crave alcoholic beverages including beer or wine?

    Enter 10 for Yes, 0 for No

14. Does tobacco smoke really bother you?

    Enter 10 for Yes, 0 for No

Enter your responses to the questions in Section 1 below:

1. _____
2. _____
3. _____
4. _____
5. _____
6. _____
7. _____
8. _____
9. _____
10. _____
11. _____
12. _____
13. _____
14. _____
SECTION 1 TOTAL _____

SECTION 2: MAJOR SYMPTOMS

Instructions:
For each symptom that is present, record the appropriate score.

- *Record a "0" if a symptom does not apply to you.*
- *Record a "3" if a symptom is occasional or mild.*
- *Record a "6" if a symptom is frequent and/or moderately severe.*
- *Record a "9" if a symptom is severe and/or disabling.*

1. Fatigue or lethargy

2. Feeling of being "drained"

3. Poor memory

4. Feeling *"spacey"* or *"unreal"*

5. Inability to make decisions

6. Insomnia

7. Muscle aches

8. Muscle weakness or paralysis

9. Pain and/or swelling in joints

10. Abdominal pain

11. Constipation

12. Diarrhea

13. Bloating, belching or intestinal gas

14. Troublesome vaginal burning, itching or discharge

15. Prostatitis

16. Impotence

17. Loss of sexual desire or feeling

18. Endometriosis or infertility

19. Cramps and/or other menstrual irregularities

20. Premenstrual tension

21. Attacks of anxiety or crying

22. Cold hands or feet and/or chilliness

23. Shaking or irritable when hungry

Enter your responses to the questions in Section 2 below:

1. _____
2. _____
3. _____
4. _____
5. _____
6. _____
7. _____
8. _____
9. _____
10. _____
11. _____
12. _____
13. _____
14. _____
15. _____
16. _____
17. _____
18. _____
19. _____
20. _____
21. _____
22. _____
23. _____
24. _____
SECTION 2 TOTAL _____

SECTION 3: ADDITIONAL SYMPTOMS

Instructions:
While symptoms in this section commonly occur in patients with illnesses having a fungal component, they also occur commonly in patients who don't. This section acts to reaffirm the results from the first two sections.

For each symptom that is present, record the appropriate score.

- *Enter a "1" if a symptom is occasional or mild.*
- *Enter a "2" if a symptom is frequent and/or moderately severe.*
- *Enter a "3" if a symptom is severe and/or disabling.*

1. Drowsiness

2. Irritability or jitteriness

3. Lack of Coordination

4. Inability to concentrate

5. Frequent mood swings

6. Headaches

7. Dizziness/loss of balance

8. Pressure above ears, feeling of head swelling

9. Tendency to bruise easily

10. Chronic rashes or itching

11. Psoriasis or recurrent hives

12. Indigestion or heartburn

13. Food sensitivity or intolerance

14. Mucus in stools

15. Rectal itching

16. Dry mouth or throat

17. Rash or blister in mouth

18. Bad breath

19. Foot, hair or body odor not relieved by washing

20. Nasal congestion or post nasal drip

21. Nasal itching

22. Sore throat

23. Laryngitis, loss of voice

24. Cough or recurrent bronchitis

25. Pain or tightness in chest

26. Wheezing or shortness of breath

27. Urinary frequency, urgency, or incontinence

28. Burning on urination

29. Spots in front of eyes or erratic vision

30. Burning or tearing of eyes

31. Recurrent infections or fluid in ears

32. Ear pain or deafness

Enter your responses to Section 3 below:

1. _____
2. _____
3. _____
4. _____
5. _____
6. _____
7. _____
8. _____
9. _____
10. _____
11. _____
12. _____
13. _____
14. _____
15. _____
16. _____
17. _____
18. _____
19. _____
20. _____
21. _____
22. _____
23. _____
24. _____
25. _____
26. _____
27. _____
28. _____
29. _____
30. _____
31. _____
32. _____

SECTION 3 TOTAL _____

Total Your Score

Simply add your scores from Section 1, 2, and 3 for your total score then compare your score with the "Understanding Your Score" section below.

Section 1 Score _____

Section 2 Score _____

Section 3 Score _____

TOTAL SCORE _____

Understanding Your Score

The Total Score will provide a strong indication as to whether you would benefit from the information in the book, *"How I Reversed My Mom's Emphysema."* Scores in women will run higher since 7 items in the questionnaire apply exclusively to women, while only 2 apply exclusively to men.

Women: 180 or higher Men: 140 or higher	It is extremely likely you would benefit from the information in the book.
Women: 120 or higher Men: 90 or higher	It is probable you would benefit from the information in the book.
Women: 60 or higher Men: 40 or higher	It is quite possible you would benefit from the information in the book.
Women: Less than 60 Men: Less than 40	Does not necessarily mean that you would not benefit from the information in the book, it just means it was not evident from the results of this test.

"When I did this test for my mother she scored a 264!"

Chapter 7: Exercise The Fountain of Youth

Exercise is one of the most important factors in maintaining health and in many cases in reversing problems that have compromised our health. I firmly believe that exercise IS the fountain of youth. No matter how long it has been, you need to get into a regular exercise program for your arms, legs, buttocks, chest stomach and back.

Walking is an excellent exercise and it is not strenuous on the joints. Swimming is extremely good for everyone. You need to decide what exercises you wish to include. Once you decide you then need to arrange to do these exercises a minimum of four times a week. Do not do more than six days a week. No matter how light the exercise, it is always a good idea to take a break from it for at least one day each week.

The one factor that researchers have found that reverses the effects of Alzheimer's Disease is exercise. Jack LaLane is around 90 and still kicking. When he was 75 he pulled 75 boats through San Francisco harbor with his teeth which is approximately 3 miles. We should all wish we were that healthy.

Make sure to include exercise as an absolute necessity in your life no matter how little of it you can do at the beginning. You just need to get started and then you can build on it over time with more time and more variety in the exercise you participate in.

Most large hospitals have a Rehabilitation Center on campus. You can usually arrange to be sent there by your doctor and your insurance company may even pay for it. If this is not an option you might want to look for a treadmill or a stationary bicycle for your house. It is easy to climb on either one of them almost every day. No traveling necessary.

I recommend having two or three options so the exercise does not become stagnant. You may want to walk one day and ride your stationary bicycle another. Maybe swim one day at the local YMCA and ride your bike with a friend or family member another. Whatever you do, make sure you include exercise in your weight loss schedule. Obviously you want to be fit and trim and looking vibrant and healthy and exercise is necessary to achieve that look and feel. I recommend weight training to greatly enhance your weight loss. You will see why in a few sections when you see the added benefits of weight training.

Warm-up and Stretching

Warming up and stretching lets your muscles know that you are planning on being active for more than just a few minutes. Letting your muscles know that this is a long-term activity causes your body to dip into its fat reserves. If you begin exercise fast and vigorous without warm-up it causes your body to use up its available sugars for energy because your body thinks it will be a short burst of activity. Warm-up and stretching are nearly as important as the exercise itself since without it your body will not be advancing toward your goal of losing fat because it will not be dipping into its fat stores.

Aerobics

Aerobics is essentially defined as any activity that involves the large muscle groups that you can sustain for at least 30 minutes. Aerobic activities include swimming, walking, running, bicycling, and dancing, just to name a few.

Ideally, if you are going to participate in aerobic activity to aid in your weight loss it is recommended that you start slowly. You can always speed up later. If you are walking you can increase the distance for a while and then maybe down the road a ways you can begin to speed up the walking.

You should perform your aerobic activities for at least 3 days a week to begin with and work your way up to 5 or maybe even 6 days. Always have at least one day for rest and recovery. If you have chosen aerobics as your exercise activity try to increase the 30 minute sessions slowly up to one hour. Remember, this is not a temporary situation it is a life changing experience. You are getting thin and healthy and making permanent changes to your life so you can stay thin and healthy! Just wait until you get your first compliment on how great you look. You will be smiling from ear to ear.

Weight Training (Resistance Training)

Weight training or resistance training is an extremely good choice for anyone wanting to lose weight simply because it not only makes you healthier but it burns a large number of calories in the process. Not to mention the fact that it continues to burn calories even after you are done with your workout. This is in addition to the fact that if you are working out on weights you are building muscle and muscle cells burn additional calories just by being there and assist you in your quest to lose excess fat.

I didn't say, "Lose Weight" here because muscle weighs more than fat. In other words, a specific volume of muscle weighs more than that same volume of fat. Muscle is denser than fat. Put some fat in water and watch it float. Put the same volume of muscle in water and it sinks to the bottom because of its added density.

This additional muscle that you build with your resistance training will also mean more enzymes and mitochondria used for burning fat. So we see that by gaining muscle we burn fat in the process and then after we build the muscle the muscle cells burn additional fat just by their mere existence.

Weight training is one very good reason why you should not worry so much about what the scale is reading today. You can actually lose 30 pounds of fat and gain 15 or 20 pounds of muscle. Your clothes are falling off of you because of the fat loss but the scale only shows 10 to 15 pounds of weight loss. It doesn't reflect the fact that you have actually lost 30 pounds of fat. You may experience a reduction in your waistline of 3 or 4 inches which does not generally accompany a mere 10 to 15 pound weight loss.

The Effect of Exercise on Fat Cells and "Set Points"

So we see that exercise is a necessary aspect to any true weight loss program. Stretching and warming up before you exercise will prepare your body to burn fat instead of starting right into vigorous exercise and burning only your available sugars. The exercise will not reduce the number of fat cells you have but it will cause them to "empty" their contents which will be used for energy to support the exercise. Your weight loss program will be successful only if you include exercise in your weight loss program as you make these global changes in your lifestyle.

Chapter 8: How Much Water is the Right Amount?

Everyone knows that water is important and that most of us need more than we drink but very few of us know how much water is the right amount. I have found many estimates as to the volume of water a human should drink but many of these benchmarks make no accommodation for the size of the person. I am sure that a 300 pound person needs more water than an 80 pound person. I therefore shy away from those stating that humans need 8-12 oz glasses of water a day or men need 13 cups of water a day and women need 9 cups of water a day. There is no way for these estimates to be accurate without taking into account the size of the person.

The best estimate I found in my research that seems reasonable is to multiply your weight by 0.66 and convert your answer to ounces. In other words, if you weigh 100 lbs. you will need to drink,

(0.66)(100 lbs) = 66 oz./day

Besides water intake, water quality is also important. In general, tap water is the lowest quality. Some well water is even lower quality with more contaminants and impurities than tap water. Depending on where you live in the country, some well water is probably cleaner and has less contaminants than other choices. Filtered water can be among the best depending on how thorough the filtering process is. Many new water filters that attach to your faucet use a 4 stage filtering system.

Distilled water is my preference. Distilling water involves boiling the water converting it to steam first and then condensing it back into liquid form. This removes impurities because the water will boil and become steam (gas) leaving behind the impurities. Once it is condensed, it is returned to a liquid state in an extremely pure form. Water distillers can be purchased from http://www.we-beat-prices.com for less than $100.

You decide what method to use but try to get away from tap water and well water unless it has been tested for impurities and harmful chemicals.

Water is so very essential to health in general. Make sure you consume the right amount and the highest quality water you can get your hands on.

Remember also that the more active and the hotter the temperature the more water you need to drink. The Israeli Army did some research in the Sinai Dessert and found that their soldiers needed one liter of water every hour while active in the dessert. This was a primary factor in them defeating the Egyptians who had depleted their water supplies and rendered their soldiers almost too weak to fight.

Try to replace other things you drink with good, clean pure water. You should not be drinking soda, sweetened tea, sweetened coffee, Kool Aid™ or punch or any other drink with sugar. Many energy drinks and even some of the "vitamin water" products have large amounts of sugar. Even many fruit drinks have added sugar. They call them "cocktails." So when you

See on the label, "Grape Juice Cocktail" you know that is grape juice watered down with sugar added. Not much of a cocktail.

You should also leave alcohol alone during the first three months on the New Menu. All alcohol, including beer and wine, are mycotoxins which are produced by fungi. Many people will tell you that, "a glass of wine each day is good for your heart." Actually, it is the resveratrol that is beneficial to your heart and it can be found at many health food stores and is contained in many foods. (See the Phytonutrients section under the *Flavonoids* listing on page 64.) The Master Formula from Primal Nutrition includes resveratrol and many other phytonutrients such as *alpha lipoic acid* and *phosphatidyl serine*.

Try to stick to water whenever you can and eliminate all sugary drinks. For the first three months don't even have honey, fruit or fruit juices. Green apples are the only fruit on the New Menu that you will be following for three months. After that you will be able to add some of the foods and drinks that you have eliminated from your diet during these first three months.

Remember when you are exercising you need additional water so always increase your water intake on these days.

Along with exercise and the New Menu, ice water will actually help you lose weight. Your body burns calories warming up the ice water. Granted, the amount of calories you burn from drinking ice water is minimal it can actually make a difference over the long haul if you are drinking the optimal amount of water.

A glass of ice water will cause you to burn an additional 15 to 20 calories. If you drink the desired amount of water you could burn as much as 75 to 100 extra calories each day which over time will make a difference. Keep in mind it is the combination of all of the factors combined that will result in successful weight loss.

Chapter 9: What the Future Holds

What the future holds is totally up to you. Staying as close as you can to the New Menu will assure the pounds don't come back and it will ensure that you stay as healthy as possible. Eating healthy is important for everyone but sometimes what we perceive as eating healthy is not. We may not realize it until we learn a little about how our body functions and what it does with the various types of food we eat.

Even though you may have lost the weight you wanted to lose, don't stop your study of healthy eating. There is a myriad of information available online that will get you eating healthier all the time. Be wary of the sites run by the pharmaceutical industry or one of their many advocates. They will denounce supplements in favor of prescription medications. They will cite studies where a synthetic form of some vitamin or other supplement was used to prove the natural vitamin or supplement doesn't work the way the supplement companies say they do. They often do studies on a vitamin or supplement and instead of using quality natural preparations they use some synthetic pharmaceutical concoction. Make sure and read between the lines when you run across these studies.

God put everything on this planet that we need to keep these bodies of ours healthy, it was no accident or happenstance. Man put the pharmaceutical companies on the planet and their primary focus is profit! Don't forget this important point.

Always check medications out before agreeing to take them. You can do a search online and just type in "side effects" after the drug name and then look for sites that are message boards where patients are writing the comments and describing what has happened to them while taking these drugs. Not a week goes by without hearing of another class action lawsuit against one or more of these pharmaceutical companies because of serious side effects one of their drugs has caused.

Cheating is a fact of life. I don't know anyone who has stuck to this New Menu without straying once or twice. I like to stray once or twice a month. I eat the food that I know is not good for me, I feel like crap the next day and I'm satisfied for another two weeks or so. When you have to cheat, cheat but don't give up and act like now that you have cheated you're a failure. Just make sure after you cheat you get right back on the New Menu. Don't beat yourself up when you cheat. Let it happen and then go back to the healthy foods but always take note of how awful you feel physically after you eat them. If you don't feel like crap after eating the unhealthy foods then you did not stay on the New Menu long enough before cheating. You need to go at least 3 months without cheating. It's difficult but you know you are worth the trouble so stick to your commitment to yourself. Remember, what you eat in private shows in public.

Cheating does not mean you are a failure. It just means you are human which is a good thing.

When I have ice cream I usually think about it for a week or so before I actually buy the ice cream. There is a shop near my house that makes their own ice cream that is absolutely to die for and they give huge scoops. When I cheat I go to this high quality, home-made ice cream shop. Don't go buy a five gallon tub of ice cream at the grocery because it is cheaper per scoop.

Don't cheat often. That is the key. If you limit cheating to once or twice a month you will do fine. I wouldn't suggest that at the beginning. Try to stay as close to the New Menu as possible for the first month. If you can, try to go 3 months at the beginning without cheating. This will also make the ill feelings that result from eating the bad food more pronounced.

When you cheat, cheat for one meal or snack. Don't cheat for the whole day. Cheating for the whole day is the best way to get back into your old habits and more disastrously, your old foods. Even if you do this because you have visitors or you are out of town or on vacation, go ahead and cheat for however long and then get back to the healthy foods.

I never thought I would lose my affinity for sweets but I have. I have been on the New Menu for about 4 years now and have totally lost my desire for them all together. I can almost make myself sick if I think about donuts and ice cream long enough. Just wait until you wake up one morning and you are hungry for a salad. It totally blew my mind when it happened to me! I didn't want to tell anyone because

I didn't want them to think I was crazy. Now here I've put it in a book!

Appendix 1

Meal Suggestions

The following are suggested meals that stay within the guidelines of the New Menu. In some cases you may not wish to eat the processed meat like bacon and ham. You may want to try turkey bacon or eliminate the meat all together. You will also notice that I have included some fruit with plain yogurt for dessert. You may want to have these fruits sparingly at first to enhance your weight loss efforts. Remember this is a new way of living and we are not robots so we will need to stray slightly from the New Menu occasionally.

Breakfast

Recipe #1
2 eggs poached or boiled
1 slice of bacon
½ green apple (or ½ grapefruit or 2 slices of tomato or avocado)

Recipe #2
2 eggs poached or boiled
1 slice of ham
½ green apple

Recipe #3
Plain organic yogurt with fresh blueberries

Recipe #4
I hardboiled egg
1/2 organic grapefruit

Lunch

Recipe #1
Marinated, baked fish fillet
Steamed broccoli
Fresh Romaine lettuce salad with tomatoes and zucchini

Recipe #2
Grilled, marinated chicken breast
Steamed fresh carrots
Fresh Romaine lettuce salad

Recipe #3
Baked Parmesan chicken
Steamed fresh green beans
Fresh Romaine lettuce salad with tomatoes and yellow squash

Recipe #4
Grilled ground sirloin or chuck burgers with chopped onions and garlic
Steamed asparagus
Fresh Romaine lettuce salad with tomatoes and white onions

Dinner

Recipe #1
Chicken or turkey salad
Tomatoes
Fresh Romaine lettuce salad with additional vegetables of your choice

Recipe #2
Stir fry organic beef and broccoli
Fresh Romaine lettuce salad with additional vegetables of your choice
Plain organic yogurt with fresh cut pineapple chunks

Recipe #3
Organic ground chuck or sirloin meatballs
Fresh Romaine lettuce salad with additional vegetables of your choice

Recipe #4
Stir fry organic chicken and carrots
Fresh Romaine lettuce salad with additional vegetables of your choice

Tasty Low Fat Recipes

The following low fat recipes are presented here with permission of http://www.dietandfitnesstoday.com. Check their web site for additional recipes and information on all aspects of weight loss.

Abbreviations:
lb - pound
tb - tablespoon
ts - teaspoon
c - cup
cl – clove
cn - can
ds – dash
pk – package
sm – small
lg – large
md - medium

Lunch or Dinner

Recipe #1

Hot 'n Spicy Beef Steaks
Yield: 4 Servings

Ingredients:

    1 1/4 lb Beef chuck eye steaks; boneless, cut 1" thick
    1 tb vegetable oil;
    1 ts chili powder;
    2 cl garlic cloves; minced
  1/2 ts oregano leaves; dried
  1/2 ts red pepper pods; crushed
  1/4 c Red wine vinegar;
  1/4 ts sugar;
  1/2 ts salt;

Preparation:
Combine oil, chili powder, garlic, oregano and red pepper pods in small frying pan; cook and stir over medium heat 2 to 3 minutes. Cool slightly. Add vinegar and sugar, stirring to combine. Place beef steaks in plastic bag; add cooled marinade, turning to coat. Close bag securely and marinate in refrigerator 30 minutes or up to 6 hours. Remove steaks from marinade and place on grid over medium coals. Grill 14 to 20 minutes for rare to medium, turning once. Season with salt. Carve into thin slices.

Preparation time: 7 minutes.

Marinating time: 30 minutes.
Cooking time: 14 to 20 minutes.

Recipe #2

Glazed Chicken in the Crockpot
Yield: 6 Servings

Ingredients:
```
   6  oz  orange juice, frozen concentrate
   3      chicken breasts; split
 1/2  ts  Marjoram
   1  ds  Ground nutmeg
   1  ds  garlic powder
 1/4  c   water
   2  tb  cornstarch
```
Preparation:
Combine thawed orange juice concentrate (not regular orange juice) in bowl along with the marjoram, garlic powder and nutmeg. Split the chicken breasts to make 6 serving sizes. Dip each piece into the orange juice to coat completely. Place in Crockpot. Pour the remaining orange juice mixture over the chicken.

Cover and cook on low for 7-9 hours, or cook on high for 4 hours if you wish. Precise cooking time is not important in Crockpot cooking. 3. When chicken is done, remove to serving platter. Pour the sauce that remains in Crockpot into a saucepan. Mix the cornstarch and water and stir into the juice in pan.

Cook over medium heat, stirring constantly, until thick and bubbly. Serve the sauce over the chicken.

Preparation Time: 8 minutes. Garlic is optional.

Recipe #3

Crockpot Turkey Breast
Yield: 2 Servings

Ingredients:
1.5 lbs turkey Breast; (boneless)
  1 pk Dry gravy mix. Chicken
  1 c   Dry White Wine
  1   onion; (Cut into four slices)
  2 sm potatoes
  2 sm Turnips
        Baby carrots

Preparation:
Cut off any fat, season with pepper and brown whole piece of turkey in skillet with olive oil. Also add onion and brown. Make sure that turkey is browned on all sides and ends. Turn with spoons, so the breast is not pricked with a fork.

Wipe the inside of the crock pot with olive oil and put carrots on the bottom, next add potatoes, turnips and onions. (I like turnips and hubby likes potatoes, so I do both) Place turkey on top of vegetables. Mix gravy with the wine and a 1/4 to ½ cup of water. Pour on top of the turkey and vegetables. Cover and cook on high for a couple of hours and then turn to low for three hours. You could put it on longer on the low setting. Just depends what your schedule is. I check every so often to make sure turkey is moist. Thicken gravy if necessary.

To Serve: Slice turkey and put gravy on top and serve with the veggies. This would serve 2-3, but the turkey does shrink, so one has to determine how large a serving they want to serve. I would suggest 4-5 ounces.

Recipe #4

Aloha Chicken
Yield: 6 servings

Ingredients:
- 2 1/2 lb chicken; pieces, skinned
- 2 chicken bouillon cubes; (Borden Low Sodium)
- 1 tb margarine
- 1 c green pepper; diced (1 med. pepper)
- 1 c radishes; thinly sliced
- 1 c pineapple, raw; chunks, canned, unsweetened
- 1/2 c pineapple juice
- 1 ts light soy sauce
- 2 tb flour

         ds pepper
 4 1/2 c   rice; cooked
           chow mein noodles; optional

Preparation:
Simmer the chicken in water with bouillon cubes. Remove meat from bones and cut into chunks. Save 1 cup of chicken broth. While chicken is cooking, melt margarine in frying pan or wok and sauté the radishes, green peppers, and pineapple until crisp tender, but not brown. (Put rice on to cook.)

Mix 1 cup saved chicken broth with ½ cup pineapple juice and 1 tsp. soy sauce. Add to pan. Mix flour with 1 Tb. cold water and stir to remove lumps. Add to vegetables. Add cut up chicken and a dash of pepper, and cook until everything is hot. Serve over rice. If desired, sprinkle chow mein noodles on top.

Recipe #5

Chicken Almond Stir Fry

Yield: 5 Servings

Ingredients:
- 1 c Chopped celery
- 1 c Chopped onion
- 1 lb Boneless; skinless chicken breasts, cut in 1/2" cubes
- 1/2 pk (10 oz.) frozen peas; thawed
- 1 cn (8oz.) sliced water chestnuts; drained
- 1/2 A bell green pepper; seeded and cut in 1/2" pieces
- 1 c water
- 2 ts Chicken bouillon granules
- 3 tb Low sodium soy sauce
- 1 ts Sesame oil
- 2 tb cornstarch dissolved in 1/2 cup cold water
- 1/4 c slivered, toasted almonds

Preparation:

In a large heavy skillet sprayed with Pam, stir fry celery and onion over medium heat until crisp-tender. Remove from skillet. Re-spray, and brown chicken over high heat, stirring constantly. Return celery and onions to skillet. Add peas, water chestnuts, red pepper, water, bouillon, soy sauce and sesame oil. Simmer 3 minutes. Stir in cornstarch mix and cook until thickened. Garnish with almonds. Serve over rice.

Recipe #6

Chicken Italiano

Yield: 4 servings
Cooking time: 20 minutes

Ingredients:
- 14 oz tomatoes; canned
- 1/2 ts basil; dried
- 1/2 ts tarragon
- 1/2 ts salt
- 1/4 ts pepper; freshly ground
- 2 ts butter; oil or margarine
- 1 garlic; clove finely chopped
- 2 lb chicken; pieces, skinned
- 2 tb parsley; chopped or 2 tsp dry
- 1/2 c mozzarella cheese; shredded

Preparation:

Pour tomatoes into container of a blender or food processor. Add basil, tarragon, salt and pepper. Puree until smooth. Melt margarine in a large frying pan. Sauté garlic over medium heat 1 minute. (or mix in 1/2 tsp garlic powder with other spices)

Add chicken pieces, sauté, turning once or twice until golden on both sides. Cover with tomato mixture. Bring to a boil, reduce heat and simmer 15 min until tender. Remove chicken and place in a warm ovenproof dish. Stir parsley into sauce and spoon over chicken. Sprinkle with Mozzarella. Place under heated broiler 1 min just until cheese melts. Or place on a microwave-safe dish and melt cheese in microwave. Or sprinkle with grated parmesan cheese and serve immediately.

Recipe #7

Sicilian Chicken
Yield: 4 servings

Ingredients:
```
    1  ts   Dried basil
    1  ts   Dried oregano
  1/4  ts   salt
  1/4  ts   pepper
    4       Chicken breasts, boneless, skinless
    1  tb   olive oil
    1       onion, chopped
    1       garlic clove, minced
   19  oz   Canned stewed tomatoes
  1/2  ts   cinnamon
    2  ts   Red wine vinegar
    2  ts   Capers, chopped -
             or green olives
             Fresh parsley, chopped
```

Preparation:
Serve with - Couscous Steamed spinach Chocolate cake with strawberries. By removing the skin from the chicken and pairing it with low-fat couscous, you can enjoy chocolate cake, too, without blowing the bank as far as fat in concerned. In this dish, chicken is

nestled in a bed of robust Sicilian ingredients, including capers and tomatoes. Combine basil, oregano, salt and pepper; sprinkle half of the mixture over both sides of chicken. In a large nonstick skillet, heat half of the oil over medium-high heat; brown chicken on all sides, about 4 minutes. Transfer to plate and set aside.

In skillet, heat remaining oil over medium heat; cook onion, garlic and remaining basil mixture, stirring, for about 5 minutes or until softened. Add tomatoes, breaking up with spoon, cinnamon, vinegar and capers; bring to boil. Reduce heat; simmer, covered, for 10 minutes or until chicken is no longer pink inside. Sprinkle with parsley.

Recipe #8

Chicken Cacciatore
Yield: 4 Servings

Ingredients:
- 1/2 cn (7-1/2 oz) tomatoes
- 3/4 c   Sliced fresh mushrooms
- 1/4 c   Chopped onion
- 1/4 c   Chopped green pepper
- 3 tb   Dry red wine
- 1   Clove garlic -- minced
- 1/2 ts Dried oregano -- crushed
- 1/4 ts salt
- ds   pepper

2	md	Whole chicken breasts Skinned -- boned & split paprika
2	ts	cornstarch
2	tb	Cold water
4	oz	Spaghetti -- cooked

Preparation:

In a medium skillet cut up the undrained tomatoes. Add mushrooms, onions, green pepper, wine, garlic, oregano, salt & pepper. Place chicken pieces on the tomato mixture in skillet. Bring to a boil; reduce heat; cover and simmer for 25 minutes. Keep warm. Combine cornstarch & cold water; stir into a skillet mixture. Cook and stir until mixture is thickened and bubbly. Cook and stir 2 minutes more. Arrange chicken and spaghetti on platter; spoon sauce over chicken.

Recipe #9

Lemon Soy Chicken

Yield: 4 servings

Ingredients:

1		Chicken, in pieces [3 lb]
1/4	c	soy sauce, low-sodium
2	tb	lemon juice
1	tb	vegetable oil
1/2	ts	Lemon pepper
1/2	ts	Ground ginger

1		garlic clove, minced
1	c	Long-grain rice
		Grated lemon rind

Preparation:
Remove skin from chicken pieces; place chicken in shallow dish. Combine soy sauce, lemon juice, oil, lemon pepper, ginger, 1 cup water and garlic; pour over chicken. Cover and refrigerate for at least 8 hours or up to 24 hours turning occasionally.

Sprinkle rice evenly in bottom of 12-cup greased casserole; arrange chicken pieces over rice. Pour in marinade. Cover and bake in 325F 160C oven for 40 minutes. Uncover; bake for 30-40 minutes or until chicken is no longer pink inside. Garnish with lemon rind.

You can substitute 2 lb chicken legs for the chicken; bake in a 13x9-inch baking dish. Lemon pepper can be found in most spice sections of supermarkets.

Recipe #10

Spanish Chicken

Yield: 1 servings

Ingredients:
- 8 Chicken legs [4 lb]
- 2 tb olive oil
- 1 tb Butter
- 1 onion, cut in wedges
- 2 garlic cloves, minced
- 3 carrots, sliced
- 1/4 c Fresh parsley, chopped
- 2 bay leaves
- 1/4 c Dry white wine, or chicken stock
- 1/4 c Pitted black olives, chopped
- 1/4 c Pine nuts
- 2 tomatoes, diced
- salt
- pepper

Preparation:
Remove skin from chicken legs. In skillet, heat and butter over medium heat; brown chicken legs in batches, if necessary. Remove chicken from skillet and set aside. In the same skillet, cook onion and garlic for 3 minutes. Return chicken to skillet along with carrots, parsley, bay leaves and wine; cover and simmer for 30 minutes. Remove bay leaves. Add olives, pine nuts and tomatoes to skillet; simmer for about 2 minutes or until heated through. Season with

salt and pepper. Arrange chicken legs and vegetables in serving platter. Serve remaining liquid separately as sauce.

Recipe #11

Braised Steak and Green Pepper
Yield: 6 servings

Ingredients:
- 1 1/2 lb   Lean steak, cut 1/4" strips
- 2 tb   All purpose flour
- 1/2 ts   salt
- 1/4 ts   Freshly ground pepper
- 1 tb   vegetable oil
- 1 3/4 c   Beef broth
- 1 c   Canned tomatoes with juice
- 1 md   onion, sliced
- 1   Clove garlic, finely chopped Or 1/2 tsp garlic powder
- 1 lg   green pepper, cut in strips
- 1 1/2 ts   Worcestershire sauce

Preparation:
Chunks of zucchini may be used instead of green pepper. Coat strips of round steak with flour mixed with salt and pepper. Heat oil in a large frying pan. Brown meat on all sides, drain off any fat. Add broth, tomato juice (reserving the tomato pieces for later), onion and garlic to the meat. Cover and simmer about 1 hour until meat is tender. Add tomato pieces, green

pepper strips and Worcestershire sauce. Stir-cook 4 to 5 minutes longer. Good served with rice.

Appendix 2

Recommended Reading

Alkalize or Die, Dr. Theodore A. Baroody. Holographic Health Press, Waynesville, NC.

The Cholesterol Myths, Uffe Ravnskov, M.D., Ph.D. New Trends Publishing, Inc.

The Fungus Link: Volume 1, 2, 3, Doug Kaufmann.

About the Author

W. G. Miller left the software industry when his mother was diagnosed with emphysema. He had worked in hospitals as a young man while attending college at Southern Illinois University and knew the prognosis was not good for emphysema patients in general. At the time she was already in End Stage Emphysema. He took a 6 month leave of absence from his software company to take care of his mother while she died.

He began to research emphysema and COPD even though the doctors said there was no way to reverse or cure emphysema. Out of desperation he began to apply his research findings and much to his surprise she began to improve. The doctors said she would not improve and her demise was eminent. She eventually went from her low of 77 pounds and on 4 liters of continuous oxygen back up to her original weight at the time of diagnosis of approximately 100 pounds. (She was only 5 feet tall)

Mr. Miller wrote his techniques, therapies and diet into a book entitled, *"How I Reversed My Mom's Emphysema."* This book is currently available at http://www.OptimalHealthProtocols.com.

Various people around the country began to write in and call stating that their spouse had gone on the diet with them and had lost weight they had not been able to lose for many years and prompted Mr. Miller to write this book on dieting to assist people in their quest for weight loss and optimal health.

As a result of this research another book is currently planned for release in January 2010 entitled, *"Get Healthy, Stay Healthy: The Optimal Health Protocols."*

The Bible says that the years of man shall be 120 years yet no one seems to be making it. This book explores why we are not living to 120 years and what we need to do to fix the problems that ultimately signal our demise. Is it the food we eat, the medications we take or the lack of exercise and water we include in our daily lives or is it possibly all of the above? Find out before it is too late! Get your copy in January!

Bibliography

American Journal of Clinical Nutrition, 2003, 76: 1308-1316

Anthony Robbins, Awaken the Giant Within (New York: Simon & Schuster, 1991), p. 185.

http://health.nytimes.com/health/guides/specialtopic/weight-anagement/print.html

http://win.niddk.nih.gov/statistics/

http://www.cdc.gov/nchs/nhanes.htm

http://www.dietandfitnesstoday.com.

http://www.faqs.org/nutrition/Met-Obe/National-Health-and-Nutrition-Examination-Survey-NHANES.html

http://www.healingwithnutrition.com/products/kyolicgarlic.htm/products/kyolicgarlic.htm

http://www.health.harvard.edu/newsweek/Glycemic_index_and_glycemic_load_for_100_foods.htm. "International tables of glycemic index and glycemic load values: 2002," by Kaye Foster-Powell, Susanna H.A. Holt, and Janette C. Brand-Miller in the July 2002 American Journal of Clinical Nutrition, Vol. 62, pages 5–56.

http://www.medicinenet.com/obesity_weight_loss/article.htm

http://www.prlog.org/10335113-obesity-global-epidemic-and-overweight-and-obesity-issues-solved-only-aastha-healthcare.html

http://www.surgeongeneral.gov/topics/obesity/calltoaction/fact_glance.htm

http://www.thecommunityguide.org/obesity/index.html

Journal of the American Dietetics Association 1995;95:791-797

Nutrition Secrets, by Charles W. Van Way, Carol S. Ireton-Jones - 2004 - Medical - 284 pages

POTASSIUM BICARBONATE ANTIDOTE TO DISEASE??, C. Norman Shealy, M.D., Ph.D., http://www.selfhealthsystems.com/archiveletter.php?id=240
European Journal of Nutrition, 2001, 40: 200-213.

www.ingramcontent.com/pod-product-compliance
Lightning Source LLC
Chambersburg PA
CBHW061508180526
45171CB00001B/87